DISASTER FIRST AID

4th Edition

What To Do When 911 Can't Come

Created in response to the urgent need for Disaster Preparedness Training at the citizen level. Includes Disaster Rapid Triage, a 24-Hour Action Plan, Emergency Care for yourself and others in the first minutes and hours of a catastrophic emergency when the most lives are either saved or lost, and a Survival Guide for the days that follow.

The information and techniques in this course are standard practices used by Disaster Response Public Safety Agencies in California and the United States, adapted to the citizen and volunteer level of ability and resources. These formulas and actions are intended for use in situations when massive emergencies make overwhelmed normal 911 Emergency and Rescue services unavailable or seriously delayed. These actions are done to preserve many of the lives that would otherwise be lost while waiting for basic essential first-care life-support measures. They are NOT a substitute for professional medical care or rescue at any time when that is available.

dfaTXT 102519

Printed in USA ISBN# 978-0-9841730-5-1
First printing 2001 Darkhorse Press, Oakland California
All book and course materials ©1996-2019

TABLE OF CONTENTS

We wish to thank the
Fire and EMS First Responders of California.
Every Firefighter, EMT, and Paramedic
has contributed
to the creation of this book
either in fact or in spirit.
For what you do day in and day out,
from the heart, Thank you.

INTRODUCTION
A Whole New Kind of First Aid

FEMA and all California Offices of Emergency Services and Emergency Management have declared that in the event of a massive multi-casualty emergency or disaster such as major earthquake, normal 911 resources will be overwhelmed. There will not be enough local help for everyone, and for the majority of people, the wait for medical help and rescue is expected to be from 24 hours to several days or longer.

Disaster First Aid© is designed for average citizens; it will enable them to respond to major emergencies with the same standard first-actions that Firefighter EMT and Paramedic First Responders use, adapted to the citizen's level of ability and resources.

This course contains the critical essentials for saving the savable lives and limbs that otherwise could be lost due to complications from waiting too long for help. The skills and information are written in clear plain language with no medical words and no unrealistic expectations. Anyone can save lives if they know these simple but critical things to do, and do them within the first minutes and hours, the time when the most lives are either saved or lost.

Disaster First Aid Rapid Triage* identifies and classifies which injured need help worst and first. This triage formula, adapted from the principles of S.T.A.R.T. Triage, has been used successfully by Emergency First Responders for nearly 40 years. It determines the priorities for you, so you don't have to decide. Recognizing life-threatening conditions and applying simple correct skills does save lives. In this course, you will learn how to identify those conditions and perform those skills.

_____

About the Author:
The creator of Disaster First Aid is a state of California Fire Service Training and Education System (CFSTES) registered Regional Fire Instructor, a former firefighter, Fire Training Officer and Emergency Medical Services Officer, Program Director of Fire Med a California EMSA approved Continuing Education Program for EMTs and Paramedics Provider #01-0022, and a Hospital Emergency Medical Technician with more than 25 years of Hospital and Field experience.

*Disaster First Aid Rapid Triage was created in 1996, adapted for citizens and non-professionals from S.T.A.R.T. Triage. The original system of S.T.A.R.T. Triage was created in 1983 by Emergency doctors and nurses of Hoag Memorial Hospital of Newport Beach California and Firefighters and Emergency Medical care providers of Newport Beach Fire Department. S.T.A.R.T. or some similar form of field triage is commonly used throughout the U.S. and Canada and many developed countries of the world.

HOW TO USE THIS BOOK

This course is intended for citizens and volunteer helper-rescuers. This Handbook is the short-form of the course. From it you can teach yourself and others the Action Plan, the formulas & skills, and how to set up a realistic first aid kit for disaster. These common-sense techniques can be learned and practiced by anyone from age 14 to seniors.

Have Fun Doing the Skills
Hands-on practice is essential and also a lot of fun. It's possible to learn these techniques by reading the book and practicing them yourself, but learning is more effective and more fun when you do it with a group. Set aside an evening or weekend afternoon, invite your neighbors and friends. Practice doing the Head-to-Toe Exam, controlling bleeding, and splinting each other's "broken bones." Follow the written information with the actual physical actions. Read, discuss, then get up and practice the things you talked about. The hands-on practice makes the learning "stick" permanently in the mind.

Get Body Wisdom
We use this hands-on method for training firefighter and paramedic first-responders because doing the actual steps and actions locks the knowledge into the neuromotor pathways of your body, so that even when the conscious mind forgets, the body remembers. In a crisis when seconds count, once the body starts moving, it knows what to do and the mind quickly catches up.

Use What You Have
In a disaster, you may not have medical supplies available, but you don't need feel helpless or intimidated by the lack of them, because you can improvise with whatever you do have. In this course you learn to adapt common items in the home or office to make dressings, bandages, and splints. Things like clean handkerchiefs, sanitary napkins, disposable diapers, or other absorbent clean materials make good dressings. Bandanas, neckties, or bedsheets torn in strips make good bandages to hold them in place. Cardboard, folded magazines or newspapers are good for splint materials, with towels or other soft materials for padding. Pillowcases, triangles cut from cloth, and even T-shirts can make good slings. We encourage "outside the box" thinking for practical problem-solving. Learn to use whatever you have, and you will always find what you need, no matter where you are. In the rest of the book there are more suggestions, a First Aid Supplies list and a diagram for making a Roll-Up First Aid Supplies kit-bag.

Plan and Teach a Class for your Community, Workplace, or School
You don't have to be a professional teacher or a medical professional to teach this course. Not only Nurses, EMTs, and Paramedics, but also coaches, camp counselors, Scout Masters, and others can teach DFA in your community or workplace group. There may often be a wide range of ages in the same class. No problem – everyone helps each other. This how it will be in a real emergency.

Police Department, Fire Department, Teachers and other professional and community educators can obtain a complete "Instructor Kit" teaching package that includes: Instructor Guide, Teaching Outline, class forms and worksheets, Task Checklist and Equipment Checklist, and detailed 80-slide color Powerpoint presentation. The Instructor i can only be purchased from the website, but the handbooks are available though any bookstore, including Barnes & Noble, Amazon, Ingram. www.disasterfirstaid.com. Or Inquire by Email: instructors@disasterfirstaid.com

Questions that may come up:

In Disaster Rapid Triage* for example, when having to "Tag" anyone, especially with a Black/ White "Deceased" or "Unsalvageable" marker. People sometimes think that they are making decisions about someone's medical care. It should be made very clear that they/you are not.

Disaster First Aid's Rapid Triage is adapted for citizens and non-professionals from the principles of fire and police service S.T.A.R.T. Rapid Triage which Medical and Rescue professionals have used successfully for more than 35 years. You are simply following the formula, knowing that this is the best chance we have to save the most lives. Statistics prove that this system is highly effective, and no special medical knowledge or medical training is needed to use it.

How Much Should You Do ?

You are never obligated to do any action that you feel unsafe, unable, or unwilling to do. It's natural to be frightened in a hazardous situation, and you should never feel that you MUST do anything. Just do what you feel you can, and remember to keep yourself safe.

What about CPR ?

CPR by itself normally cannot save the life of someone who has no breathing and no heartbeat. Except for extremely rare instances, CPR must be followed with the "Chain of Survival" which includes defibrillation, Hospital ER, intravenous medications, cardiac monitoring, possibly surgery, and 24 hours in a hospital ICU. This process must start within minutes. Usually this person must receive professional medical care within 10 to 20 minutes in order to have a chance of survival, some or all of which will be impossible in a massive disaster when hospitals are overflowing and there are not enough beds or ambulances to respond immediately to all of those who need help. Hospitals must prioritize for those who have a reasonable chance of survival, which is very different from a normal, non-disaster, with only a "one patient at a time" situation.

You should certainly attempt CPR if you believe help might be available. And ALWAYS open the airway to assist breathing. Sometimes that may be all that's needed to save a life. Unfortunately, sometimes there are circumstances that are beyond our human limits, and the harsh reality is that there may be some we cannot help.

ACTION OUTLINE: the first 24 hours

This is the STANDARD SYSTEM OF DISASTER RESPONSE used by Public Safety agencies, Emergency Medical, Paramedic, and Fire Dept/ Rescue. In this Disaster First Aid course the system has been simplified and adapted to the citizen's level of ability and resources.

1. SIZE-UP: the area and situation. Check YOURSELF for injuries. DON'T rush in, Stop and LOOK. What hazards are there? Are YOU safe ? Move into the open and look for a Safe Area.

2. TAKE CHARGE: Say in a loud voice "EVERYONE WHO IS ABLE TO WALK, GET UP AND MOVE TO (your chosen safe area near by). These are the "walking wounded" people with minor injuries or none. You will now rapidly TRIAGE all the ones who DID NOT WALK. You will use some of the walking wounded as helpers to assist you.

3. **RAPID TRIAGE and TAG:** Use the Rapid Triage system. Begin with the hurt person nearest to you and move from one to another. Do not enter areas that seem unsafe. Do only the specific treatments of the Rapid Triage System. As you Triage, you will MARK the injured: Red-Immediate or Yellow-Delayed or Black/White-Unsalvageable or Deceased. The walking wounded will be marked later as Green/Minor (least priority).

4. REQUEST HELP: Send a messenger to the nearest Fire Station with this information:
    a. Your exact location (including nearest cross-street)
    b. Any hazards, such as fire, gas leaks, or building collapse.
    c. How many Serious, Moderate, and Minor injured you have, and if any deceased.
    d. The approximate total number of people at your location.
Later you will send more information. Right now, do not wait to gather more than these basic facts, and deliver them to your local Communications Network and get on the list for help.

5. HEAD-TO-TOE EXAM: Go back to the injured that you have Triaged and tagged or marked. Start with the worst first (Red-tag/ Immediate) and examine each person for injuries. Write down their names and what the injuries are. Also write health information such as pre-existing medical conditions, medications they take regularly, and any allergy to medications. Next you will examine the Yelow-tag/Delayed-tagged ones.

6. TREATMENT: Send your SECOND REPORT to the Fire Station. Then treat the injuries you found, as time allows before help comes. Treat for shock, clean and bandage wounds, splint and immobilize suspected fractures.

7. GATHER and PLAN: Make provisions for water, shelter, bedding, food, and sanitation.

8. IN THE DAYS THAT FOLLOW: Protect yourself and others from the dangers of infection, disease, and exposure hazards of heat and cold.

That's the WHAT – Now let's look at HOW > > >

TRIAGE: do the most good for the most people

Disaster First Aid Rapid Triage is adapted from the principles of S.T.A.R.T. triage* a system used by Fire Dept. and Paramedic First Responders throughout the U.S. This simple formula quickly detects potentially life-threatening conditions and provides critical first-actions. Rapid Triage is designed for multi-casualty situations and intended to be used by both professionals and non-professionals. The purpose of Triage is to quickly identify those who need help first and give the most critical and/or life-supporting treatments as soon as possible to prevent worsening or death.

Professional Rescuer First Responders use a special Triage Tag to identify the injured by color-code and category which is easily recognized by other Rescuers when they arrive. The injured persons marked "Immediate" having a RED tag will be looked at first for treatment and transport to a medical facility; the YELLOW tag "Delayed" people will be helped next.

You can buy Triage tags or tapes or use the copyable Triage Tag in this book. Or you can use whatever you have, to mark each individual as you triage them. You can use plain colored tags or tape (red, yellow, green, black) or write the word "Immediate" "Delayed" "Minor" or "Deceased" with a marker in an obvious place, such as upper arm or forehead.

*The system of S.T.A.R.T. Triage was created in 1983 by Emergency doctors and nurses of Hoag Memorial Hospital of Newport Beach California and Firefighters & Emergency Medical care providers of Newport Beach Fire Dept.

To begin your Rapid Triage

Speak in a loud voice. Tell everyone who is able to Get Up and Walk to a safe place near by that you direct them to. Those who do get up and move, have now identified themselves as "Minor" not needing immediate urgent treatment. These "walking-wounded" will be green-tagged after the more critical are tagged and treated. For now they can act as your helper-pool.

Now Triage all who did NOT get up and walk
WHAT THE CATEGORIES MEAN:

"I" for "Immediate" (Red tag)
Means rapid medical treatment is necessary because of possible life-threatening injuries or conditions such as shock, breathing problems, uncontrolled bleeding, serious head injuries, etc.

"D" for "Delayed" (Yellow tag)
Means these injuries are more than minor but are not life-threatening. Some examples might be sprained ankle, possible broken arm, bruises, minor bleeding that has been controlled.

"M" for "Minor" (Green tag).
These are the "walking wounded" with only minor injuries or none, and will be tagged last after triage is done. You can use them to assist you as Helpers and Messengers.

"U" for "Unsalvageable /deceased" (Black / White tag or write "DECEASED" on whatever tag.)
Those with massive irreversible injuries, or else not breathing after you open their airway.

TRIAGE: tags and other markers

You can use the Met-Tag Public Safety personnel use, or the copyable Triage Tag in this book, or use colored labels, tags, or triage tapes. Or if you have nothing else, use a Magic-marker or even a lipstick to mark on the forehead of the injured person: "IMMEDIATE," or "DELAY" or "UNSALVAGEABLE," whatever you find.

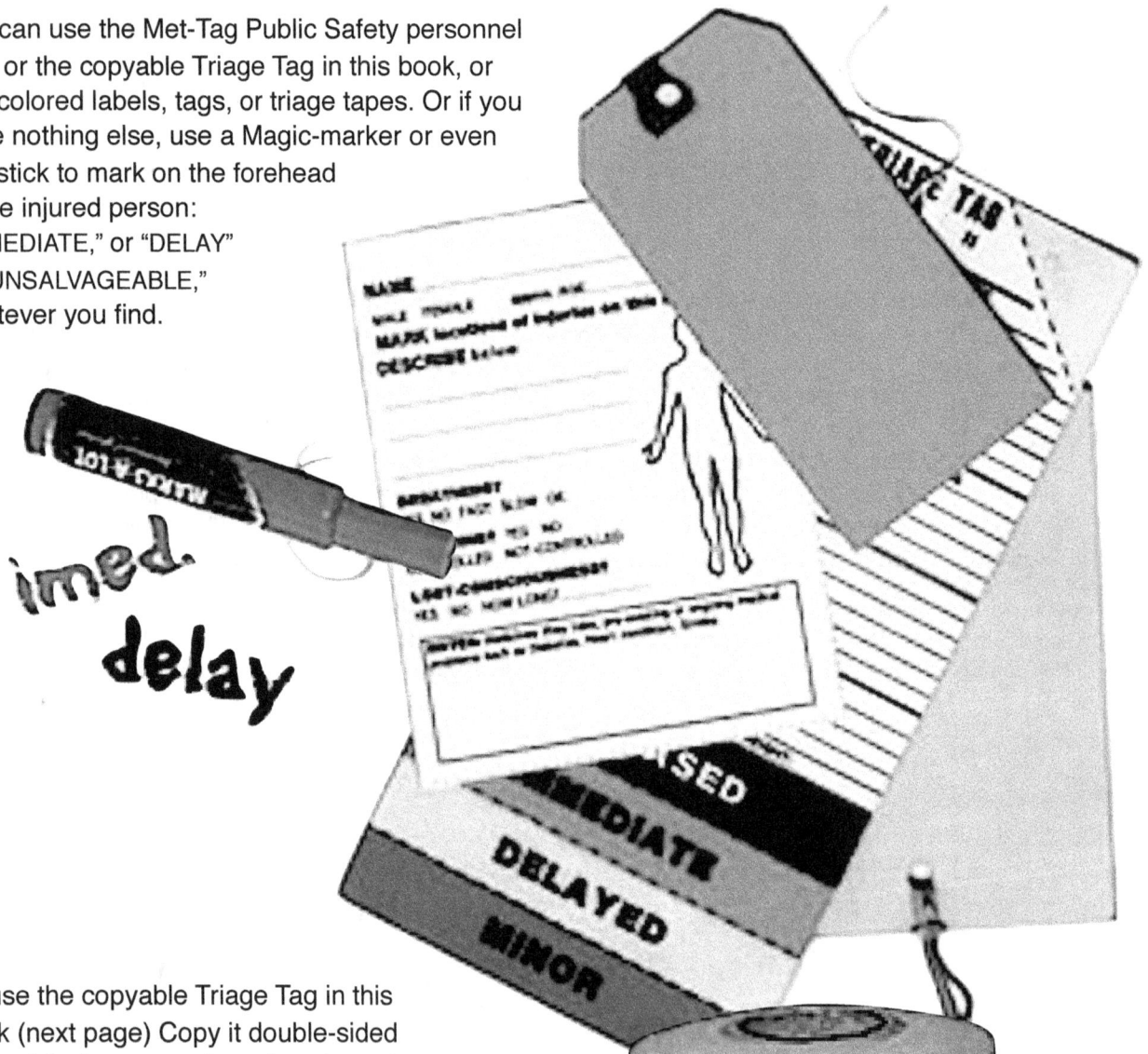

To use the copyable Triage Tag in this book (next page) Copy it double-sided onto white heavy card-stock, cut apart into individual tags, hole-punch and add string or a large safety pin.

As soon as all the injured have been triaged, marked, and given the first level of Triage-Treatments, SEND A MESSENGER to the nearest Fire Station with your **First Report**.

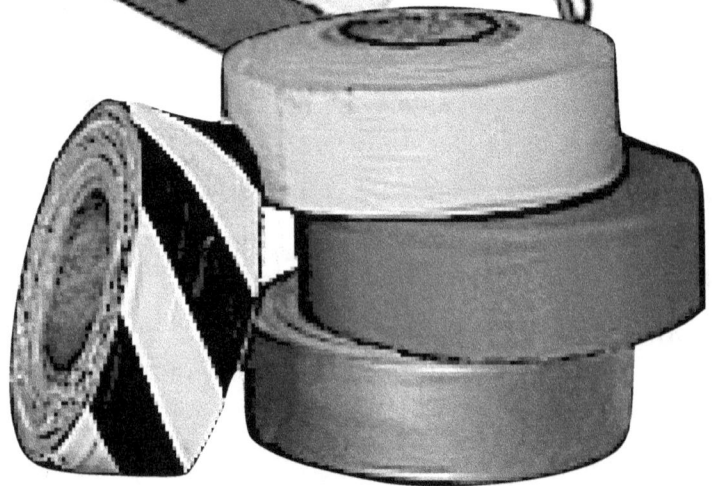

THIS SIDE FIRST

☐ RED-TAG / immediate IF

○ At Checkpoint **1-BREATHING**
is Faster than 30 breaths per min. OR
stopped breathing then re-started. OR:

○ At Checkpoint **2-CIRCULATION**
No pulse at wrist, but still breathing. OR

○ At Checkpoint **3-MENTAL STATE**
unable to follow simple commands, answer
questions, or unconscious. OR

○ ANY INJURY YOU BELIEVE TO BE
LIFE-THREATENING

☐ YELLOW-TAG / Delayed IF - - -

This person **PASSED ALL 3 CHECKPOINTS**
and although injured, does not appear to be
life-threatened. (When in doubt, use RED tag)

AFTER all injured are TRIAGED & MARKED
GO BACK to each one, do HEAD-TO-TOE exams,
and fill out the other side of this Tag.

THIS SIDE FIRST

☐ RED-TAG / immediate IF

○ At Checkpoint **1-BREATHING**
is Faster than 30 breaths per min. OR
stopped breathing then re-started. OR:

○ At Checkpoint **2-CIRCULATION**
No pulse at wrist, but still breathing. OR

○ At Checkpoint **3-MENTAL STATE**
unable to follow simple commands, answer
questions, or unconscious. OR

○ ANY INJURY YOU BELIEVE TO BE
LIFE-THREATENING

☐ YELLOW-TAG / Delayed IF - - -

This person **PASSED ALL 3 CHECKPOINTS**
and although injured, does not appear to be
life-threatened. (When in doubt, use RED tag)

AFTER all injured are TRIAGED & MARKED
GO BACK to each one, do HEAD-TO-TOE exams,
and fill out the other side of this Tag.

THIS SIDE FIRST

☐ RED-TAG / immediate IF

○ At Checkpoint **1-BREATHING**
is Faster than 30 breaths per min. OR
stopped breathing then re-started. OR:

○ At Checkpoint **2-CIRCULATION**
No pulse at wrist, but still breathing. OR

○ At Checkpoint **3-MENTAL STATE**
unable to follow simple commands, answer
questions, or unconscious. OR

○ ANY INJURY YOU BELIEVE TO BE
LIFE-THREATENING

☐ YELLOW-TAG / Delayed IF - - -

This person **PASSED ALL 3 CHECKPOINTS**
and although injured, does not appear to be
life-threatened. (When in doubt, use RED tag)

AFTER all injured are TRIAGED & MARKED
GO BACK to each one, do HEAD-TO-TOE exams,
and fill out the other side of this Tag.

THIS SIDE FIRST

☐ RED-TAG / immediate IF

○ At Checkpoint **1-BREATHING**
is Faster than 30 breaths per min. OR
stopped breathing then re-started. OR:

○ At Checkpoint **2-CIRCULATION**
No pulse at wrist, but still breathing. OR

○ At Checkpoint **3-MENTAL STATE**
unable to follow simple commands, answer
questions, or unconscious. OR

○ ANY INJURY YOU BELIEVE TO BE
LIFE-THREATENING

☐ YELLOW-TAG / Delayed IF - - -

This person **PASSED ALL 3 CHECKPOINTS**
and although injured, does not appear to be
life-threatened. (When in doubt, use RED tag)

AFTER all injured are TRIAGED & MARKED
GO BACK to each one, do HEAD-TO-TOE exams,
and fill out the other side of this Tag.

Head to Toe EXAM   PUNCH HOLE

NAME _____

MALE   FEMALE   Date of Birth_____ or Age

MARK locations of injuries on this outline
and describe below:

_____

_____

_____

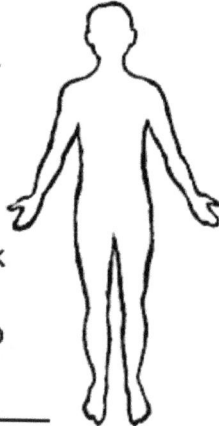

BREATHING?
YES /NO FAST/SLOW OK/NOT OK

BLEEDING? YES / NO
CONTROLLED / NOT-CONTROLLED

LOST-CONSCIOUSNESS?
YES / NO For How Long? _____

NOTES: Medicines they take, pre-existing or ongoing medical
problems such as Diabetes, Heart condition, Stroke, other.

Head to Toe EXAM   PUNCH HOLE

NAME _____

MALE   FEMALE   Date of Birth _____ or Age

MARK locations of injuries on this outline
and describe below:

_____

_____

_____

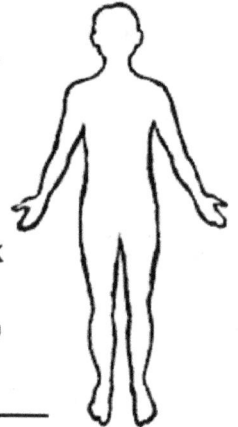

BREATHING?
YES /NO FAST/SLOW OK/NOT OK

BLEEDING? YES / NO
CONTROLLED / NOT-CONTROLLED

LOST-CONSCIOUSNESS?
YES / NO For How Long? _____

NOTES: Medicines they take, pre-existing or ongoing medical
problems such as Diabetes, Heart condition, Stroke, other.

Head to Toe EXAM   PUNCH HOLE

NAME _____

MALE   FEMALE   Date of Birth _____ or Age

MARK locations of injuries on this outline
and describe below:

_____

_____

_____

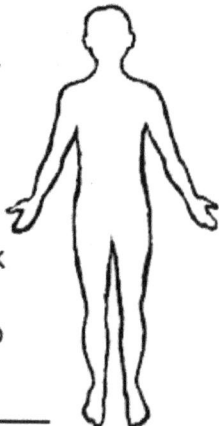

BREATHING?
YES /NO FAST/SLOW OK/NOT OK

BLEEDING? YES / NO
CONTROLLED / NOT-CONTROLLED

LOST-CONSCIOUSNESS?
YES / NO For How Long? _____

NOTES: Medicines they take, pre-existing or ongoing medical
problems such as Diabetes, Heart condition, Stroke, other.

Head to Toe EXAM   PUNCH HOLE

NAME _____

MALE   FEMALE   Date of Birth _____ or Age

MARK locations of injuries on this outline
and describe below:

_____

_____

_____

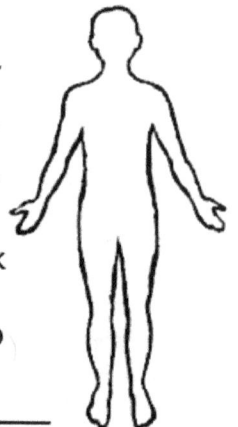

BREATHING?
YES /NO FAST/SLOW OK/NOT OK

BLEEDING? YES / NO
CONTROLLED / NOT-CONTROLLED

LOST-CONSCIOUSNESS?
YES / NO For How Long? _____

NOTES: Medicines they take, pre-existing or ongoing medical
problems such as Diabetes, Heart condition, Stroke, other.

Simple Triage and Rapid Treatments

ONLY 3 TREATMENTS:

1. **OPEN** •the AIRWAY
2. **CONTROL** •visible BLEEDING
3. **POSITION** •Recovery Position: Turn the person on their SIDE and prop in position.
   •Shock Position: Raise legs & feet 10 to 20 inches above heart level.
   •Head Injury: Raise the head – not the legs. (See Positioning p.19)

Rapid Triage identifies critical factors so they can be treated quickly. When you find the FiRST FAILED checkpoint, TAG, TREAT, and MOVE ON to the next person. Wear rubber gloves if possible and protect yourself from blood or body fluids as best you can.

ONLY 3 CHECKPOINTS:

1. BREATHING

Is breathing NORMAL? (quiet,12 to 24 breaths per min.)
If MORE than 30 breaths per minute- Red-tag "Immediate"
... *and move to the next person.*
If **NOT BREATHING** - OPEN the airway
If breathing now STARTS, Red-tag Immediate.
If it DOES NOT START, Black/White-tag "Deceased"
... *and move to the next person.*
IF BREATHING is OKAY - Do Checkpoint #2

2. CIRCULATION

If NO PULSE can be FELT **at wrist,** Red-tag "Immediate"
Control any bleeding. Elevate the legs quickly if possible,
... *and move to the next person.*
If CIRCULATION is OKAY - Do Checkpoint #3

3. MENTAL STATUS

Can they Follow simple commands ?
(Like: "Squeeze my hand" or "Blink your eyes.")
Can they **answer simple questions** ("What year is it?)
IF NOT, or if unconscious, Red-tag "Immediate"
Turn them onto their side (Recovery Position)
... *and move to the next person.*
IF THEY PASS ALL 3 Checkpoints -
Yellow-tag "Delayed" ... *and move to the next person.*

✱ **RED tag = Immediate/Serious.** Should be given at FIRST FAILED Check-point. Once you give a Red-tag and the Triage-treatment is done, NO MORE Check-points are done at this time. MOVE TO the next person.

✱ **YELLOW tag = Delayable/ Not severe.** Only given this status after ALL 3 CHECKPOINTS have been passed

✱ **BLACK/WHITE tag = Deceased** (or) **Unsalvageable.** NOT BREATHING even after opening the airway.

✱ **GREEN tag = Minor or Uninjured.** These will be checked too, but last, after the more serious are tagged and treated.

AFTER TRIAGE is done, you will return to the RED-TAGGED first to do Head-To-Toe Exams.

TRIAGE: Doing Checkpoint #1-Breathing

Breathing is always highest priority. With any injured person, always check the airway and breathing FIRST. If breathing cannot be established and maintained, nothing else and no amount of effort can save that person without the ability to breathe on their own.

Head injuries often cause temporary unconsciousness. Because an unconscious person becomes completely limp and loses their "gag reflex" it's possible for the tongue to fall back into the throat and block the air passageway. By quickly opening the airway and keeping it open so the person can breathe, you may save their life. When someone is breathing okay but is unconscious, turn them on their side and prop them. The tongue will naturally fall away from the throat so fluids or secretions can drain away. That way the person will not choke or suffocate or inhale fluids into their lungs.

If any injured person is NOT breathing, OPEN THE AIRWAY with the head-tilt/ chin-lift method. Place the palm of one hand on the person's forehead, and the fingers of your other hand under the bony part of the chin. To open the airway tilt the chin upward while pressing back on the forehead.

Check for breathing: Look, Listen, and Feel

Ask yourself 2 questions:

1. Is the person breathing? Lean close for a few seconds to hear and feel. Yes? or No?
2. Is the breathing normal - and enough?

   •Normal breathing QUALITY is relaxed and effortless, quiet and without pain.
   •Normal breathing RATE for adults is 12 to 24 complete breaths per minute.
   •in + out = one breath. Children and infants normally breathe faster than adults.

If not breathing: OPEN the airway. If breathing STARTS, Red tag "Immediate," turn the person onto their side, and move to the next person.

If breathing does not start: White/Black tag/ Deceased, and move to the next person.

Noisy or difficult breathing: If conscious, place them in their position of comfort. Sitting up or reclining may make breathing easier. Loosen tight collars or pants. Red-tag "Immediate."

Very fast breathing: Red-tag/Immediate.

Gurgling sounds: may mean fluid or blood in the air passage. Turn the person on their side to allow fluids to drain. Red-tag " Immediate."

Snoring or "crowing" sounds: may mean obstruction such as the tongue, or swelling. Re-open the airway. Turn them on their side. Red-tag "Immediate."

Changes in skin color: very pale, or blue, or mottled may indicate lack of oxygen. OPEN the airway, Red-tag "Immediate," and move to the next person.

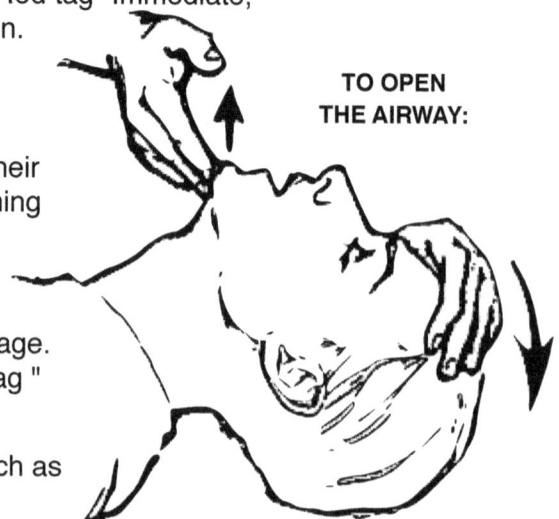

TO OPEN
THE AIRWAY:

TRIAGE: Doing Checkpoint #2-Circulation

We check Circulation (also called perfusion) to look for early signs of shock. The normal circulation of blood carries oxygen and nutrients throughout the body, brain, and vital organs. Every cell of the body must receive this constant oxygen supply in order to live.

When shock begins to occur, the body tries to survive by shifting circulation away from the arms and legs and toward the internal organs, heart, and brain, where it's needed most. This is why the arms, hands, and feet become very cool or "clammy" and skin color becomes pale or "ashen." The heartbeat becomes fast and the wrist pulse very weak. That's why we check circulation by feeling for a WRIST pulse in Rapid Triage (NOT the neck as in CPR.).

Blood loss is one cause of shock. In an adult, loss of about one quart of blood is life-threatening. Children and infants have much less total volume of blood than adults, so the loss of a much smaller amount (such as a teacup) could be serious. Always control visible bleeding. (p.21) Another cause of shock may be internal bleeding with injuries from blunt objects, falls, or crush injuries. Any injuries of the abdomen or chest, or suspected fractures of large bones could have serious invisible blood loss internally. Anyone with such injuries should be treated for shock. Always treat any suspicion of shock to prevent or decrease it before it takes hold.

To CHECK: Feel the WRIST pulse

1. **If you CAN FEEL** a strong pulse at the wrist, this person has passed checkpoint #2 – Go on to checkpoint #3

2. **But if you can CAN NOT FEEL a pulse,** or the pulse is very weak or too rapid to count, may be an early sign of shock. Red-tag "Immediate," do the appropriate Rapid Triage treatments,
   –and move to the next person.

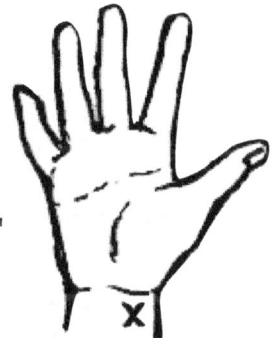

The Rapid Triage Treatments for shock are:

1. Control any visible bleeding.
2. Have them lie down. Elevate the person's legs 10 to 20 inches higher than their heart level.
3. Have someone sit with them if possible to calm and reassure them.
4. If they are unconscious or semi-conscious, make sure their airway is clear and open.
   Turn them on their side (to drain secretions or possible vomiting) and prop them in position.
   ... and move to the next person.

Altered or abnormal mental states can have many causes. Although sometimes they are not life-threatening, often an altered mental state can be a sign of an unseen serious problem. Some causes may be: shock (of any origin) head injury, lack of oxygen, hyperventilation, (breathing too fast and getting too much oxygen) Hyper- or hypothermia, too high or too low blood-sugar (sometimes found in individuals with diabetes) or other imbalances of blood chemicals, including overdose of (or lack of) drugs or medications. In Rapid Triage Checkpoint #3 we are checking for possible life-threatening conditions. We may not know exactly what the injury is, we just need to recognize the signs and take action.

What do Altered Mental States look like?

Altered Mental States in adults may be actions, emotions, or lack of emotions that are unusual or inappropriate for the situation, such as a strange silence, aggression, combativeness, confusion, forgetfulness, or repeating the same phrase over and over. Or possibly drowsiness, semi-consciousness, or complete loss of consciousness and coma.

When a child or infant is hurt or frightened, their normal response is crying. So when an injured infant or young child is very silent or strangely groggy and sleepy or seems "not like themselves" these could be signs of possible head injuries or shock. Infants and small children are more vulnerable to head injuries than adults.

To CHECK for Normal vs. Altered Mental Status:

1. ASK QUESTIONS: For example, "What is your name?" "Where are you right now? "What year is this?" "Who is the President of the United States?"

2. GIVE SIMPLE COMMANDS: such as "Squeeze my hand." "Open your eyes." or "Blink your eyes twice if you can hear me." or "Wiggle your toes."

3. With children or infants NOTICE whether they are behaving in an unusual way,

If the person is awake, alert and ABLE to answer such questions correctly, or to carry out simple commands, they have now passed Checkpoint #3 and can be Yellow-tagged or marked "Delayed." This means they are second-priority for care and transport to a medical facility when that becomes available. Tag or mark them –and move to the next person.

But if the person is UNABLE to pass this checkpoint (or any previous checkpoint) or you think their mental state is altered and not normal for them, they should be Red-tagged or marked "Immediate." (NOTE: If they seem violent or may hurt you, do not attempt to engage them. Just notice this and mark it on your triage tag. –and move to the next person.

You will return to those who need more help AFTER you Triage, Tag, and Treat ALL of the injured.

Rapid Triage and Treatment does two crucial things:

A. It discovers and marks those persons with the most serious or at-risk injuries, so you and other helpers, rescuers, and emergency medical personnel can quickly know who needs care first.

B. It gives you (as the helper/rescuer) the opportunity to quickly perform the simple first-actions and treatments that have been proven to save the most lives:

ONLY 3 Checkpoints: (Every time) **+** **ONLY 3 Treatments:** (As needed)

1. Breathing
2. Circulation
3. Mental Status

1. Open Airway , Assist Breathing
2. Control Bleeding, elevate legs to prevent Shock
3. Position injured person for safety/ recovery.

As soon as you find a FAILED Checkpoint, TAG, TREAT, & MOVE to the next person.

You can help wherever you are, because you can do these same first-actions that professional EMS responders would do. When they do arrive, they will recognize your markings, re-check all of the injured, and follow-through with the rest of the appropriate emergency medical care. Of course some of the injured will need more care than you can give them, but you will have done the most crucial things in these first few minutes, and this will give them a better chance of survival and recovery. After you have done RAPID TRIAGE on all of the injured and given the Triage treatments, you will send a FIRST REPORT with that information to get help. Then you and your helpers or "walking-wounded" will return to the red-tagged "Immediate" individuals to do a HEADTO-TOE EXAM and give further care as needed. Then you'll do the same for the Yellow-tagged. The "walking wounded" will be looked at last, but everyone should be looked at for injury.

REVIEW OF CATEGORIES

Green / Minor: At the beginning of Triage, this group of patients are moved to a separate area by rescuer ordering "Everyone who can walk..." followed by directions to go to a specific area close by, to be used as helpers when possible.

Red / Immediate: When Breathing is faster than 30 breaths per minute, OR Breathing only starts after opening the airway, OR wrist pulse cannot be felt, OR the patient is unable to correctly answer simple questions and follow simple commands.

Yellow / Delayed: This group, due to injury or other reason, did not walk to the area for minor injuries when directed to, but they passed all 3 Triage checkpoints.

Black / Deceased: No Breathing is present, even after opening the airway.

(from Alameda County California Emergency Medical Services Policy & Procedures Manual, policy #8073 S.T.A.R.T. Triage)

There is a Disaster Plan at every level of government. FEMA is the Federal agency, O.E.S. Offices of Emergency Services are set up at state, county, and city levels. It takes time to organize, gather, and distribute needed supplies and services. The numbers of injured persons will be much larger than the normal amount of 911 personnel, supplies, and services can handle at once. Therefore all help, personnel and resources will be prioritized and directed through an E.O.C. (Emergency Operations Command Center) and sent first to the areas where the need is greatest. Help may not arrive for your area for a period of several hours or days, and in some areas possibly weeks. As soon as your Rapid Triage is done, deliver your First Report information to the Disaster Response Network.

FIRST REPORT:
As soon as your Rapid Triage is done, send a runner/ messenger to the nearest Fire Station

As part of the local Disaster Response plan, "Ham" radio operators will go to Fire Stations, where they will maintain the radio communications network to relay the information to the Emergency Operations Command Center about what types of resources are needed in each area. Local O.E.S. agencies will mobilize their Disaster Response plan and start the process of organizing and distributing the needed services and supplies. Your message to the Fire Station is the fastest and most reliable link to these services.

STAY OFF THE TELEPHONE !

DO NOT CALL 911 to report a major emergency such as tornado or earthquake – They will already know. And please, NEVER call 911 for information! That wastes precious time and blocks out other communication that may be critically important. INSTEAD have a portable radio with extra batteries, pre-set the dial to the Emergency Radio station in your area. That is your best source of updated information.

Most cell-phones and land-line phones will not be working. Even if they are, the lines will be needed for emergency Police and Fire operations communications. If you must use your cell phone, use text messaging instead of voice. Text is more likely to transmit because it is a smaller electronic file. THE BEST and most effective choice is to have a pre-arranged Contact Person outside of your area that you have given your important phone numbers to. If a massive emergency or disaster happens, you will make ONE phone call to them, and they will make all other calls to your family members, employers etc. to let them know you're okay.

Out-going phone lines from inside the area will be blocked for Emergency Agencies to use, but calls originating from outside the disaster area, coming in, will be more likely to get through.

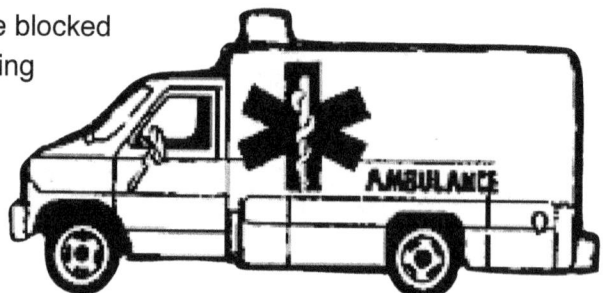

*Make TWO copies of this form to keep in your First Aid Bag along with pens and markers.

FIRST REPORT FORM

As soon as your Rapid Triage is done
send a messenger to the NEAREST FIRE STATION
with this information.
Make and Keep a Copy at your location.

Our LOCATION is _____
The CROSS STREET
(or nearest Major
street or Landmark) is: _____

The CONTACT PERSON at this site is: _____

The number of **RED-tag (immediate) SERIOUSLY injured is:** _____

The number of **YELLOW-tag (delayable) Moderate injured is:** _____

The number of **Black / White-tag (deceased) is:** _____

The approximate **TOTAL number of people at our site is:** _____

HAZARDS at our location are:

☐ Building collapsed   ☐ People trapped   ☐ Fire burning

☐ Gas leaking   ☐ Other (Describe Below)   ☐ None

HEAD-TO-TOE EXAM: Looking for injuries

After Rapid Triage has been completed and you have sent for help, go back to fully examine and treat everyone. Do the exam BEFORE moving the person if the area is SAFE to do so. First are the Red-tagged "Immediate," then the Yellow-tagged "Delayed" people. Finally, check the walking wounded. Get enough people to help you, before attempting to move someone. Avoid handling blood or body fluids. Wear gloves if available. Examine the injured person from head-to-toe without stopping to treat injuries or apply splints until you've got the "whole picture."

EXCEPT: If you find an AIRWAY problem, uncontrolled BLEEDING, or SHOCK. These hopefully were seen duringTriage and given the critical treatments then, but situations could have changed. Treat immediately if needed, just as you did in your Rapid Triage. After the Head-to-toe exam, if there are several people injured, set up a TREATMENT AREA and carefully move the injured there. Choose a place that's safe, in an open area that is accessible for ambulances and Rescue vehicles.

How to do the Head-to-Toe Exam
if possible, wear rubber or vinyl gloves to protect yourself from blood and body fluids.

1. TELL THE PERSON what you're going to do. "I'm going to examine you for injuries." If they refuse or appear combative, DO NOT insist. Move on to the next person. YOUR SAFETY always comes first. You cannot help others if you are injured trying.

2. START AT THE HEAD and work your way down to the feet. Ask them "Where does it hurt?" You look at and "palpate" (gently feel) all areas for pain response or other signs of possible injuries.

3. LOOK before palpating. Give the person as much privacy as you can, but if you suspect an injury, you will open, remove, or cut away clothing as necessary to see the injured area.

4. YOU ARE LOOKING FOR bleeding, bruising, bumps, dents, or deformities. On limbs, compare both the right and left for sameness or changes. Also look for Medic-Alert bracelet or necklace.

5. To PALPATE - Gently feel and/or press on each part as you examine it. Don't pull or twist. Feel for lumps or deformity. Watch and listen for signs of pain.

6. FEEL for PULSE and warmth at both wrists and both feet. Notice whether the pulses are: (1) present (2) strong or weak (3) fast or slow (4) equal on both right & left sides.

7. MAKE NOTES of what you find as you examine. Get the person's name and medical information and write it on the "2nd Report /Treatment Record" Form (or plain paper) and also on the Triage Tag or some other note that stays attached to the person.

8. SET UP A MEDICAL AREA If you have several injured, move them together to a central "M.A.S.H." type Medical tent or area. After you have determined what the injuries are, you can do more treatment, like cleaning and bandaging wounds, immobilizing and splinting suspected fractures, and making the injured persons more comfortable.

9. SEND a messenger to the Fire Station with a list of basic information with names and injuries. KEEP the Treatment Record in your Medical Area until Rescue or Medical Aid comes to take over care of the injured. Then give them all the information you and your helpers have gathered.

DISASTER FIRST AID ©

2nd REPORT - Triage and Treatment Record

Make 6 or more copies of this form and keep them in your First Aid bag, along with pens and markers.

DATE

LOCATION

TEAM LEADER or FIRST AIDER

Radio frequency and channel OR cell phone #

NUMBERS OF INJURED	PAGE#
RED immediate =	
YELLOW delayable =	
GREEN minor =	
BLACKorWHITE dead =	

PRIORITY	NAME + DATE OF BIRTH	AGE	SEX	PROBLEM OR INJURY	NOTES	TIME
☐ Immediate ☐ Delayable ☐ Minor			☐ M ☐ F	☐ Breathing ☐ Bleeding-Circulation ☐ Mental State ☐ Shock ☐ Fracture ☐ Other	Medications they take, any allergies to medicines, their medical history.	
☐ Immediate ☐ Delayable ☐ Minor			☐ M ☐ F	☐ Breathing ☐ Bleeding-Circulation ☐ Mental State ☐ Shock ☐ Fracture ☐ Other	Medications they take, any allergies to medicines, their medical history.	
☐ Immediate ☐ Delayable ☐ Minor			☐ M ☐ F	☐ Breathing ☐ Bleeding-Circulation ☐ Mental State ☐ Shock ☐ Fracture ☐ Other	Medications they take, any allergies to medicines, their medical history.	
☐ Immediate ☐ Delayable ☐ Minor			☐ M ☐ F	☐ Breathing ☐ Bleeding-Circulation ☐ Mental State ☐ Shock ☐ Fracture ☐ Other	Medications they take, any allergies to medicines, their medical history.	
☐ Immediate ☐ Delayable ☐ Minor			☐ M ☐ F	☐ Breathing ☐ Bleeding-Circulation ☐ Mental State ☐ Shock ☐ Fracture ☐ Other	Medications they take, any allergies to medicines, their medical history.	
☐ Immediate ☐ Delayable ☐ Minor			☐ M ☐ F	☐ Breathing ☐ Bleeding-Circulation ☐ Mental State ☐ Shock ☐ Fracture ☐ Other	Medications they take, any allergies to medicines, their medical history.	

Recognize Possible SHOCK

Early signs of shock begin quietly; they are easy to miss. Always be on guard for signs of shock, and treat preventively. Don't be distracted by blood or broken bones; be aware that there may be worse injuries that are hidden. **Anticipate shock** with any major injury, crush injuries, severe bleeding, or when there is pain or bruising to the chest, abdomen, pelvis, or large areas of limbs. Shock is always high priority.

Shock can be worsened by pain or fear, however when recognized and treated in the early stages, incipient shock can sometimes be decreased or even reversed by simple measures. Elevating the legs, maintaining body warmth, and calming and reassuring the injured person may prove to be life-saving techniques.

What Does Shock Look Like?

In various stages of shock a person may show several or any combination of these signs:

• Fast shallow breathing	•Weakness, dizziness, feeling faint
• Pale or ashen gray complexion	• Nausea or vomiting
• Cool "clammy" skin, cold sweats	• Extreme thirst
• Very fast pulse, very weak pulse or you cannot feel a wrist pulse	• Restlessness or agitation
• Unresponsive infant or silent pale child	• Mental state is altered or inappropriate
	• Decreasing level of consciousness or loss of consciousness

What to do when you suspect shock

1. Have the person lie down.

2. Elevate the legs to above their heart level. If there is a head injury, elevate the head also.

3. Protect the airway, especially if the person is nauseous, vomiting, or loses consciousness. If so, TURN them onto their side in the "Coma / Recovery Position"

4. Conserve body heat with a sleeping bag or blankets over and also under them. Cover their head with a hat, scarf or towel. Insulate them from cold ground or floor with a layer of bedding, rugs, cardboard, crumpled newspapers, dry leaves or whatever you have available.

5. Calm and reassure them. Have someone stay with them.

6. They may be very thirsty. Do not give them anything to eat or drink (to prevent vomiting and possibly aspirating fluids into lungs).

7. SEND FOR MEDICAL HELP immediately. Anyone who is in shock or appears to have serious blood loss or severe injury is HIGH PRIORITY.

POSITION the injured:

One of the 3 Rapid Triage Treatments is POSITIONING. Use whatever you have available to prop and stabilize the position, such as boxes, blankets, overturned chair, backpack, sleeping bag.

FAINTING or SIGNS OF SHOCK: elevate the legs. This sends more blood flowing to the brain and vital organs. Cover the person with blankets both over and under, and also cover the head to preserve normal body warmth.

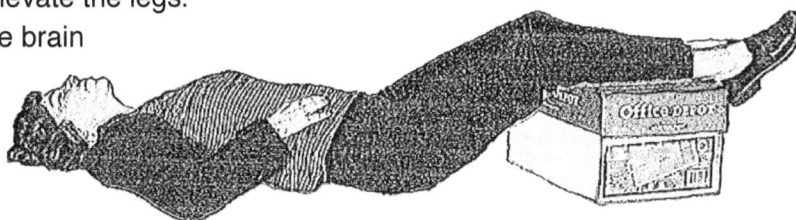

HEAD INJURY, SHORTNESS of BREATH, or DIFFICULTY BREATHING: Raise the upper body and head. This sends LESS blood to the brain, which could be important if there is a possibility of internal bleeding inside the head. With shortness of breath, breathing is often easier sitting up. Be sure to prop them so that they bend at the HIP, NOT at the chest or neck.

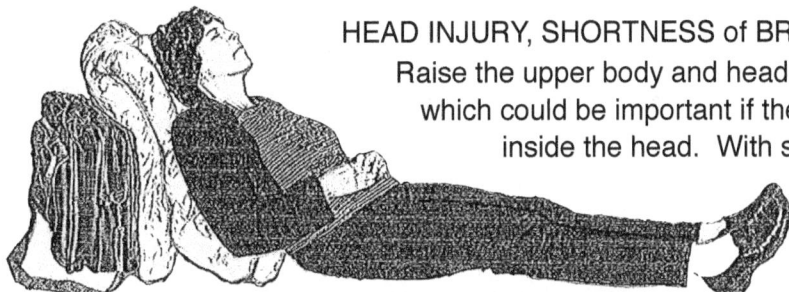

If there are MIXED SIGNS:
Like Shortness of breath combined with signs of shock,
or Head injury combined with signs of shock,
raise both the upper body and the legs.

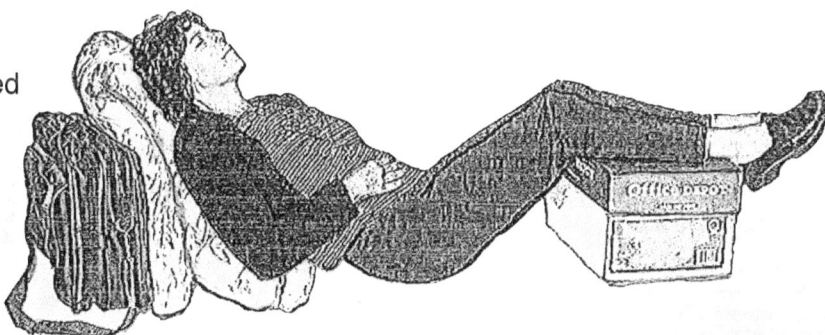

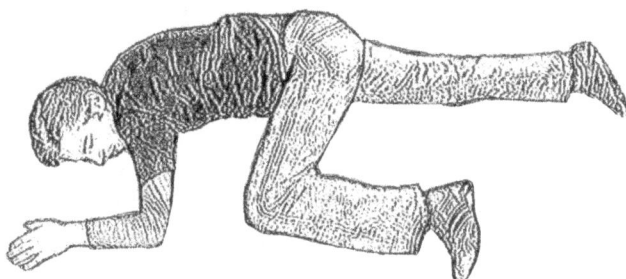

SEMI-CONSCIOUS, UNCONSCIOUS or VOMITING Use the "Recovery / Coma" position. (On their side and propped in place) This will drain fluids naturally, keep the breathing passage open, and protect the lungs from inhaling fluids.

WOUNDS: Cuts and Bruises:

Open wounds are lacerations, cuts, tears, punctures, and some burns (when skin is broken). Most open wounds bleed freely. Use the bleeding control techniques of direct pressure and elevation. After the bleeding has been controlled, clean and bandage the wounds.

Puncture wounds are made by a penetrating object such as a nail, sharp stick, flying glass. Punctures have a small opening at the surface but may be deeper than they look. They may not have surface bleeding, but may be bleeding inside. A puncture wound found on the belly, chest or neck should be given high priority. Anticipate shock and treat for it. All open wounds are vulnerable to infection. Clean and bandage the wound.

Closed wounds are bruises/contusions. They can be minor or major. Bruising often accompanies other injuries, though the "black and blue" color may not appear till later. Elevate the injured area and apply ice pack if available. If bruises and scrapes are found on the belly, chest, or neck, be suspicious of deeper injury and consider shock.

The main dangers of open wounds are excessive bleeding and infection. Punctures have less danger of external bleeding but higher risk of infection. All head, scalp, and facial wounds normally bleed more freely than other areas, but bleeding can usually be controlled with direct pressure.

With a head injury watch for changes in mental state, and always consider the possibility of brain injury, neck injury, or spinal injury. If there is any LOSS OF CONSCIOUSNESS, this person is high priority. Secure and support the neck if you can (p.28) and carefully elevate the upper body not the legs. If NOT conscious, place in "coma/recovery position" on their side to protect the airway.

With open wounds, in the next few days, watch for signs of INFECTION such as: redness, heat, swelling, pus, fever, increasing pain, red streaks up the arm or leg. Infection raises the priority.

Control Bleeding

Most surface bleeding is venous, because the arteries are deeper in the body where they are more protected. Bleeding from veins flows smoothly or seeps. Bleeding from arteries comes in spurts, in the rhythm of the heartbeat. Arterial bleeding is more dangerous and harder to control. Wear rubber or vinyl gloves if possible. Protect yourself from blood or body fluids as well as you can.

Methods for bleeding control (can be used in combination) are: (1) Direct Pressure, (2) Elevation, (3) Pressure Bandage, (4) Arterial Pressure-point. IF ALL of these FAIL after proper application, or IF there is severe, rapid, or "pumping" bleeding, (5) Apply an Arterial Tourniquet. If you do, write on the person's forehead: "TK" and the DATE and TIME it was applied.
IMPORTANT NOTE: This is not the kind of tourniquet nurses use for taking blood samples for tests or donating blood. The emergency tourniquet is intended to stop almost all circulation to everything beyond it. This means those areas now become at great risk for permanent damage due to lack of blood circulation.

Unless the bleeding is obviously extreme, try the OTHER METHODS FIRST. When used correctly, 10 to 15 minutes without peeking under the bandage, direct pressure and elevation will control 99% of bleeding you're likely to encounter. Severe or uncontrolled bleeding is HIGH PRIORITY.

TO CONTROL BLEEDING

1. With a clean cloth, apply DIRECT PRESSURE to the wound. This stops the bleeding flow and helps the blood to clot (the body's way for sealing leaks in its circulation system). Raising the wound higher than the person's heart-level decreases blood flow to it, which also aids the clotting function.

2. Hold pressure firmly and continuously for 10 to 15 minutes. DO NOT TAKE THE CLOTH OFF to see if bleeding has stopped! (That will re-start the bleeding again!) If blood soaks through the cloth, don't remove it, just add more cloth on top. If holding continuous pressure is not possible (as when you are doing Rapid Triage) get a helper to hold pressure, or tie a pressure bandage.

3. PRESSURE BANDAGE: Tie a snug band around the wound dressing and limb to hold pressure. DO NOT tie anything tightly around the neck or chest!

Pressure bandage and elevation plus arterial pressure point.

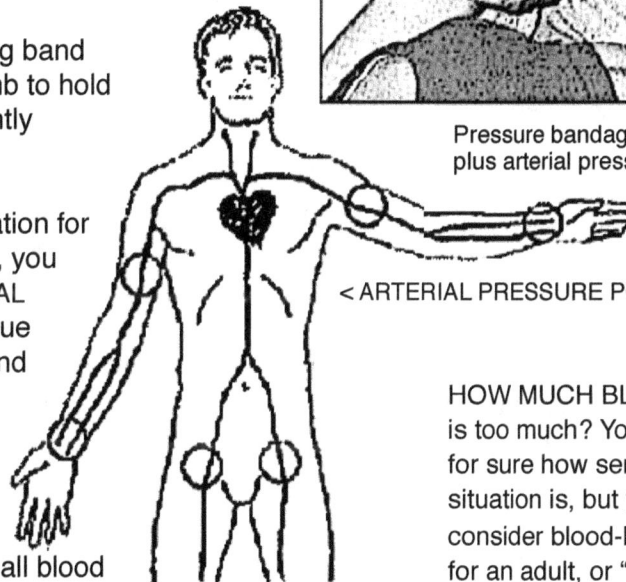

4. If continuous pressure and elevation for 15 minutes do not control bleeding, you can try firm pressure to an ARTERIAL PRESSURE POINT while you continue holding direct pressure on the wound also. Hold for another 10 to 15 minutes. Whenever you have serious bleeding, it's important to get medical help ASAP.

< ARTERIAL PRESSURE POINTS

HOW MUCH BLEEDING is too much? You can't know for sure how serious the situation is, but you should consider blood-loss of a "quart" for an adult, or "a teacup" for an infant, as life-threatening.

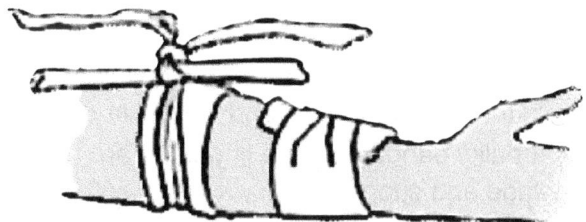

5. A TOURNIQUET shuts off almost all blood flow from both veins and arteries. When the bleeding is "spurting" or "pumping" this is arterial bleeding. Do not hesitate to use a tourniquet. Just be aware that any bleeding so severe will need medical help as soon as possible, and act accordingly.

Complications from using a tourniquet are significant. Some injuries treated with tourniquets have had amputations of limbs attributed to the use of the tourniquet. But when it's truly needed and the choice is between possible loss of limb or loss of life, the tourniquet does have great value in emergencies.

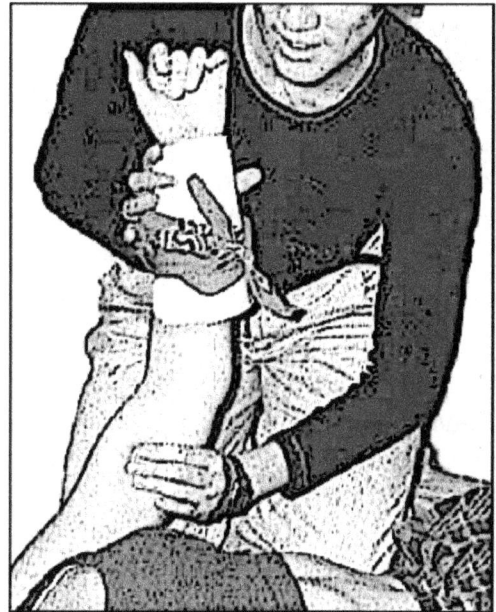

Tie the tourniquet close to the wound, between the wound and the heart. Write "TK" and the date and time on the person's forehead.

Fractures, Sprains

These may appear very similar, with pain or tenderness, swelling, and pain with movement. When there is loss of movement or severe pain during movement, always take fracture precautions and immobilize and splint the injury. This decreases pain and helps avoid further injury. A splint should support the limb at the point of injury and also at the joints above and below the injury. Fractures are more serious than sprains but the First Aid is similar for both. Fractures have the potential for more internal bleeding, swelling, and damage to nerves and tissues, especially fractures of large bones such as the thigh, hip, or pelvis. With these, anticipate shock and treat for it.

What To Do

Handle the part gently with as little movement as possible. Immobilize it with well-padded splints, leaving the fingers, if an upper limb injury, or toes if a lower limb, exposed to allow for periodically re-checking circulation by color, feeling, and movement. Raise and prop or support the injured part if it's practical to do so, to reduce swelling and pain. Apply cold packs if available. Make sure that circulation is not being impaired by your splint. Splint ties should be re-checked and may need to be loosened or adjusted over a period of time, since swelling may increase. Make the person as comfortable as you can, have them rest quietly, and prevent them from becoming chilled.

Dislocations

An odd-looking distorted limb could indicate either a fracture or a dislocation. Dislocations occur at joints (a bone forced out of its normal position) while a fracture may show itself as an unnatural lump, bend, or distortion at any point on a bone, including joints. Compare both right and left sides of the body for sameness vs. distortion. Many fractures are not visible at all from the outside.

What To Do

If you suspect either a dislocation or a fracture, carefully immobilize and secure the injury with well-padded splint materials. DO NOT try to straighten it. A dislocation is usually very painful and the injured person will be holding or guarding it, and may not allow anyone to touch it. A good splint for a dislocation is a pillow or folded blanket, secured with tape, cloth wraps, or a sling.

If the injury is to a hand, place a soft object such as a roll of cloth or ball of cotton in the palm to hold the fingers relaxed and curved in a natural position,then wrap the whole hand gently with a soft bulky bandage. If the fingertips are not injured, leave them showing. If the fingers are injured, include and support them with your soft bandage.

In general, you would Leave fingers (or toes if a lower limb injury) exposed so you can periodically recheck circulation (by color, numbness, or coldness) and signs of infection. Apply cold packs if possible, make the person as comfortable as you can.

Burns

FIRST DEGREE or "superficial" burns look like a bad sunburn. The skin is red, hot and dry. This type of burn is usually not serious in adults but can be dangerous or even life-threatening to small children and infants if large areas of skin are involved.

SECOND DEGREE burns are the most painful. There will usually be blistering and if the skin is broken the burns will seep watery fluid. If there are blisters that have not broken, DO NOT open them. Try not to break them, because keeping the skin intact helps prevent infection.

THIRD DEGREE burns are the most serious. The skin may feel hard and leathery. The burns may look white and ashy, or dark and charred. Severe burns may extend through all layers of skin, to muscle, even bone. These burns may actually be less painful than some second-degree burns because the feeling nerves have been destroyed. Third degree burns are always high priority.

Possible Other Dangers

SMOKE INHALATION: Someone who has been in a closed area with smoke or fire may develop coughing or hoarseness. Swelling in the throat and air passages could cause serious breathing problems. They should be Red-tagged "Immediate" as high priority. Watch carefully for worsening.

OTHER HIGH PRIORITY SITUATIONS: Burns to the face, hands, feet, or genitals are high priority. Burns to children and infants are high priority because they are at greater risk than adults for shock, hypothermia, and dehydration from fluid loss.

ELECTRICAL BURNS: DO NOT TOUCH the person until you are absolutely sure the electrical source is shut off and completely removed from touching them. Electrical burns and lightning burns are often more serious than they look. When an electric current has passed through a part of the body, there will be an entrance wound and an exit wound with deep tissue damage between the two. Electrical burns are high priority.

What to do
As always, quickly check breathing and circulation first.
If possible, wear rubber gloves to protect yourself from blood or body fluids.

1. Halt the burning process by applying clean cool water or water-soaked cloths for 10 to 20 minutes. Be careful not to over-chill the person.

2. Cut away and remove burned clothing. Remove jewelry before swelling starts.

3. DO NOT break blisters.

4. DO NOT apply oils, lotions, or disinfectants.

5. Cover the burns with dry sterile or clean dressings and bandage loosely.

Crush Injury

Suspect crush injuries whenever someone has been squeezed or caught between hard surfaces or under heavy objects. If the chest or abdomen are involved there may be damage to vital organs with internal bleeding that is not visible from the outside. Even when only a limb is involved, there may be extensive damage to bones, tissue, and blood vessels.

What does a Crush Injury look like ? There may be cuts, scrapes, or surface bleeding in addition to deeper damage. There may be swelling, bruising, purple or mottled coloring, with or without any surface bleeding. Sometimes crush-injured persons may show little or no visible sign on the outside. Often the best indicators of possible crush injury are severe pain and "Mechanism of Injury" (what happened to them that caused the injury).

Dangers of crushing injuries include tissue damage, possibility of nerve damage, loss of circulation to some areas, possibility of internal blood clots which can get stuck in a major vein or artery cutting off circulation, and/or possibility of internal bleeding and shock. Always suspect shock and treat for it preventively: keep the person quiet, lying down, and maintain adequate body warmth. Multiple injuries, severe pain, or signs of shock make this person HIGH PRIORITY.

Crush Syndrome

This becomes a factor when someone has been crushed or trapped for a period of time. The pressure of the crushing object itself may be blocking-off circulation and bleeding. Then when the pressure of the object is removed, the backed-up circulation starts again with greater force.

Problem: Sudden release of the pressure can release serious bleeding internally and externally. BEFORE you attempt to free the person from entrapment, PREPARE. Gather what you'll need to control bleeding (p.21) and treat for shock. (p.18) Get enough people to help.

Problem: Normal blood circulation constantly filters and removes toxins and waste products from the body. Crush injury interferes with this process. Over a period of time, toxins from damaged tissue collect and build up to dangerous levels. When circulation is restored, large amounts of toxins and wastes from the injured areas begin to travel to the heart, lungs, liver and kidneys, which can cause organ failure. Exertion will speed up that process, so the crush-injured person should be kept very quiet, calm, and still.

What to do - General

Handle any crush-injured person very gently and carefully. Do not allow a crush-injured person to get up and move around. Anticipate shock and take preventive treatment measures. Even if they look okay have them sit or lie down and remain quiet. Keep them comfortably warm. Do not allow them to assist with other rescue efforts. If possible, have someone stay with them to calm and reassure.

What to do for Crush Injury

Keep the person quiet, warm enough, and as comfortable as possible. Anticipate the possibility of shock and treat for it, especially if there is bruising or injury to the chest or abdomen. Control any external bleeding, clean and dress wounds. Persons with large or significant crush injuries or severe pain should be Red-tagged "Immediate."

If the injury is to a limb, immobilize and elevate it to decrease swelling and pain. For these injuries, swelling is dangerous and damaging. Apply cold packs if possible. Be very cautious about anything that wraps or ties around the injured limb, because it may impair circulation especially when the swelling increases. Re-check the person and the injuries periodically. To prevent the strangulation of the limb by bandages or splints getting too tight, re-check, loosen, and re-tie them as needed.

Releasing an injured person from crushing objects

If people are entrapped under rubble or debris, you must first make the decision whether or not to try to free them yourself with only other citizens to help. Sometimes it's better for untrained persons not to attempt a complex rescue.

If you decide to attempt rescue, several things must be considered, such as the amount of difficulty, time, tools, and strength needed to do the job. Get trained Search and Rescue help if you can. If that is not possible and you decide to attempt the rescue, take care for your own safety as you follow these basic guidelines.

Help the most-helpable first, the easiest to reach, with the best chance of success. In disaster the rule-of-thumb is: "Do the most good for the most people."

Preparation: Get enough help, personnel and equipment BEFORE you begin. Plan your actions. Assemble the supplies you will need so that you can treat wounds and shock immediately when the person is freed. Above all, Don't get hurt yourself.

Actions: Start at the top of the debris and work your way down, piece by piece. Large pieces that can't be removed entirely MUST be shored-up or secured in place to prevent falling and danger of further injury to the injured person or to rescuers.
– Locate all limbs before moving. DO NOT PULL on any part you can't see all of, because you may accidentally do more damage to an entangled limb. Handle the person very gently.
– If possible, splint or support all of the body and limbs before moving the person. Consider using a plank, shutter, door, coffee table, or ironing board as a makeshift stretcher.

•**Follow-up:** Carry the person carefully to a safe area. Treat for shock. Treat surface wounds and splint any suspected fractures. Calm and reassure. Have someone stay with this person continuously to monitor their condition and inform you of any changes. Signs of shock or change in mental status make this person HIGH PRIORITY.

Splinting & Immobilizing

ARM or WRIST magazine or newspaper splint. Use a small towel or other soft material for padding the splint wherever it touches the skin. Elevate the limb and secure it with a triangle sling or improvised sling. Re-check circulation to the fingers (color, feeling, movement) after splinting.

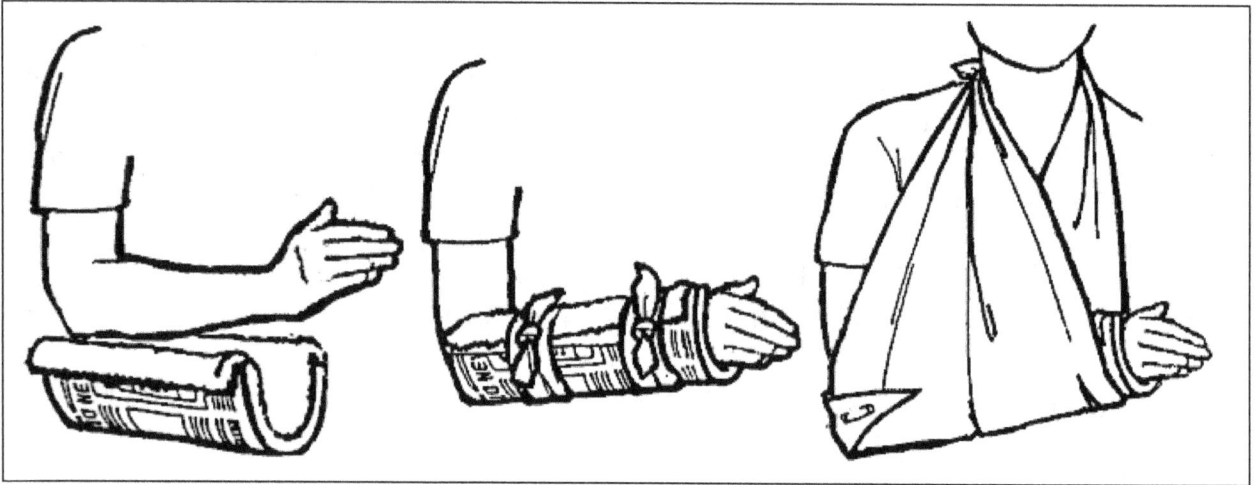

LOWER LEG or KNEE: Use a board, heavy corrugated cardboard folded over 3 times, or whatever suitable material you find available. Be sure splints are well-padded wherever they touch the skin.

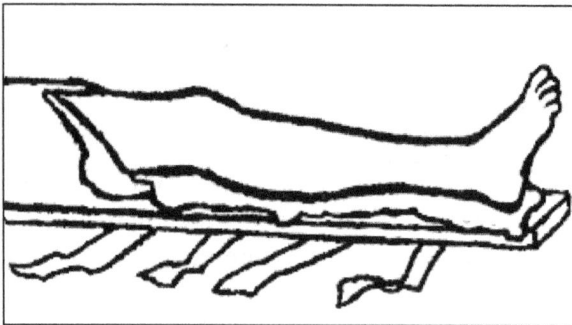

Tie the support strips to one side so that the knots will not press onto skin. Remember to check and then re-check circulation to the toes, before and after splinting the injury.

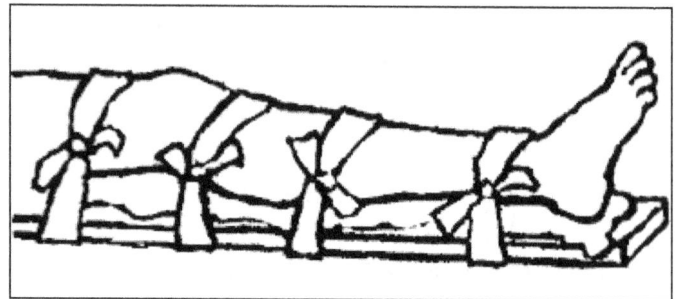

GENERAL for most closed injuries, if possible, elevate the injury and apply cold packs to the injured areas 10 to 20 minutes at a time for the first few days to reduce swelling and pain.

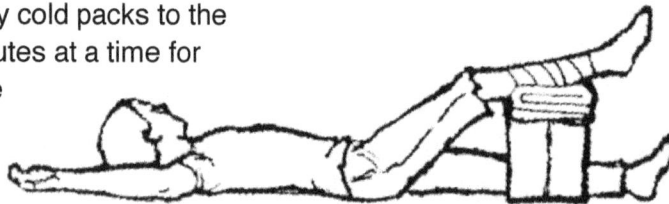

Splinting & Immobilizing

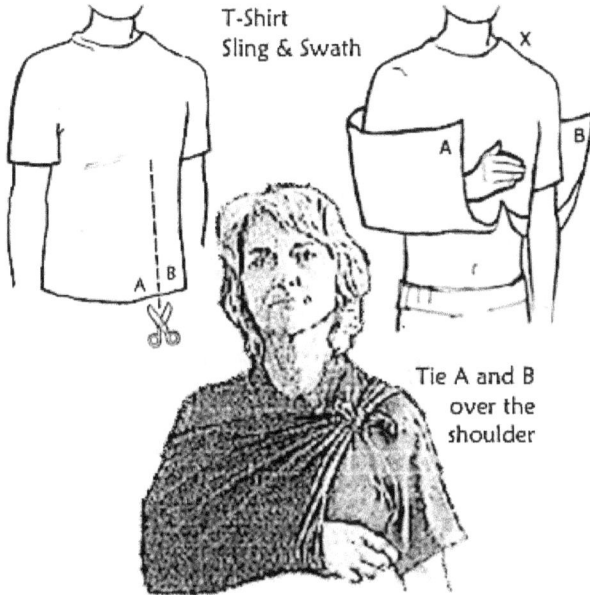

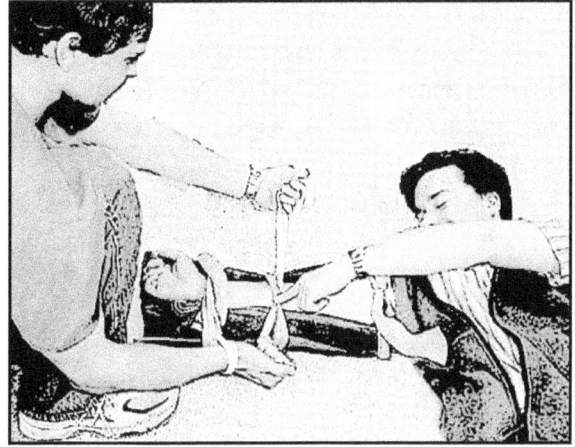

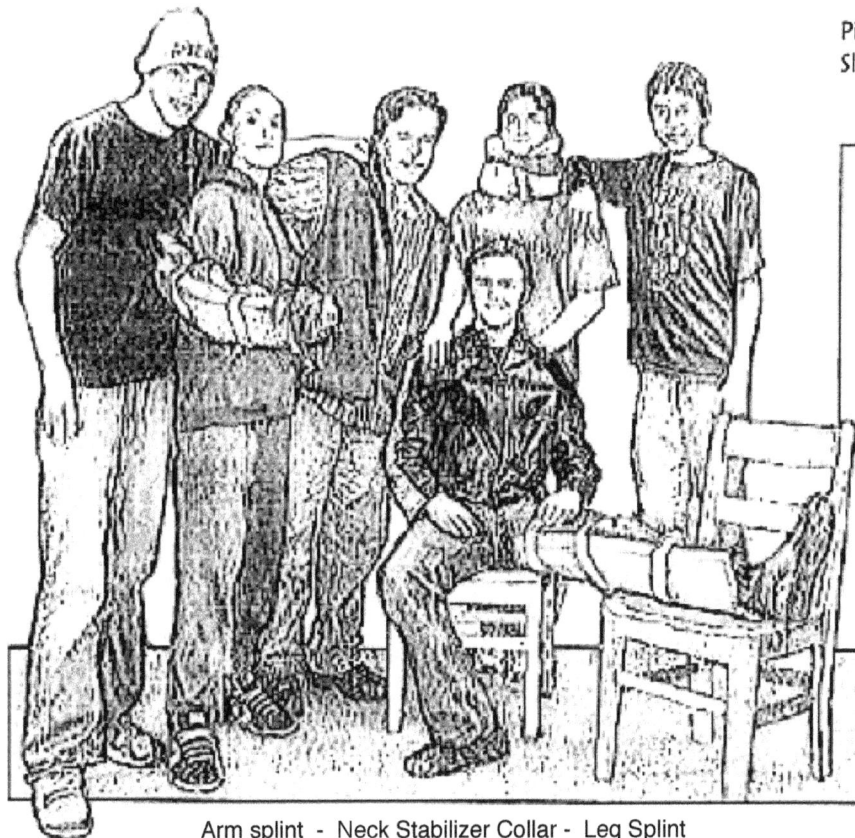

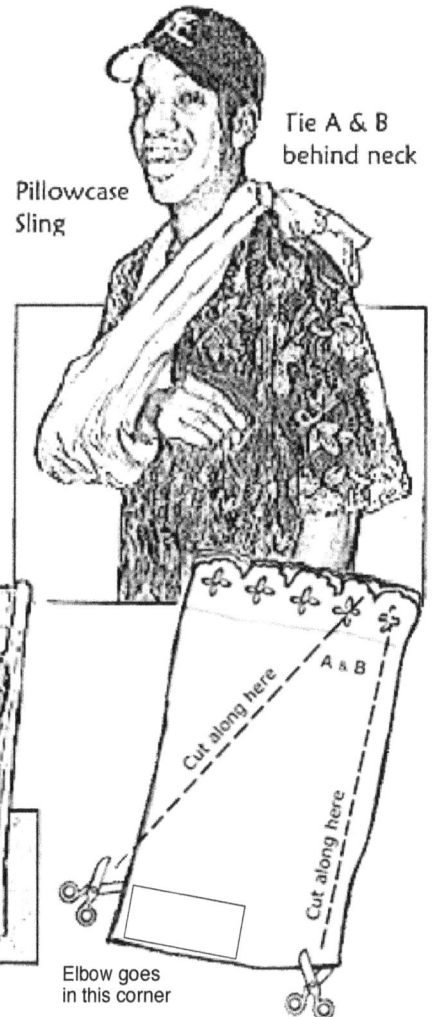

T-Shirt
Sling & Swath

Tie A and B
over the
shoulder

Wrist and forearm splint

Tie A & B
behind neck

Pillowcase
Sling

Arm splint - Neck Stabilizer Collar - Leg Splint

Cut along here

A & B

Cut along here

Elbow goes
in this corner

27

Moving the injured

If a NECK or SPINAL injury is suspected, or if the person is unconscious or has a serious head injury. One rescuer holds the head and neck in a straight alignment with the body and spine. The second rescuer or helper carefully slips a folded towel (or some other FIRM material) beneath the neck to make a wide supportive collar, and tapes it securely in place.

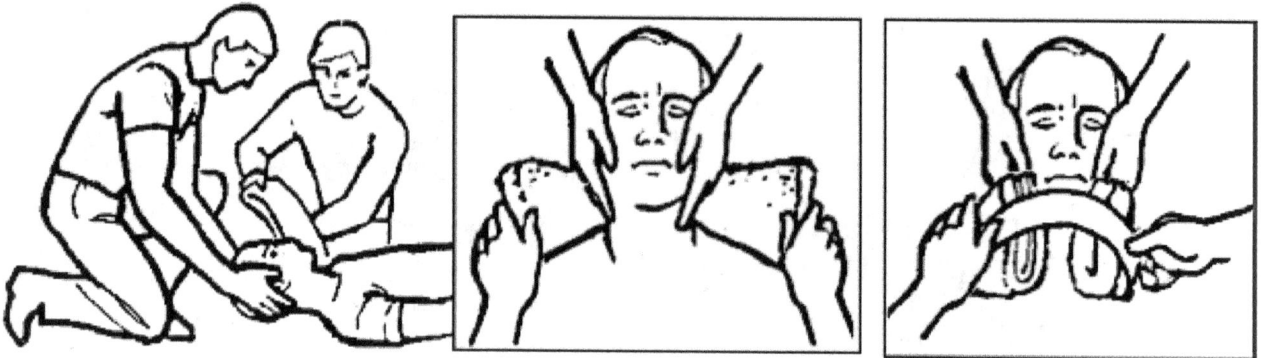

LOG-ROLL: The first rescuer continues to support the head and neck in a straight line with the body and spine. On signal (such as "Move on three – Ready? One, two, three.") all helpers together as a team ROLL the injured person onto his side, while keeping the spine straight like a log. A board or blanket can now be placed next to the injured person. Then carefully roll him back onto it, while still maintaining a straight neck and spine alignment at all times. If a carrying-board is available, Secure the injured person to the board with tape or strong ties. Then it can be lifted and carried like a stretcher. If no board is available, a blanket can be used to carry them or to carefully drag them in a straight line like a sled.

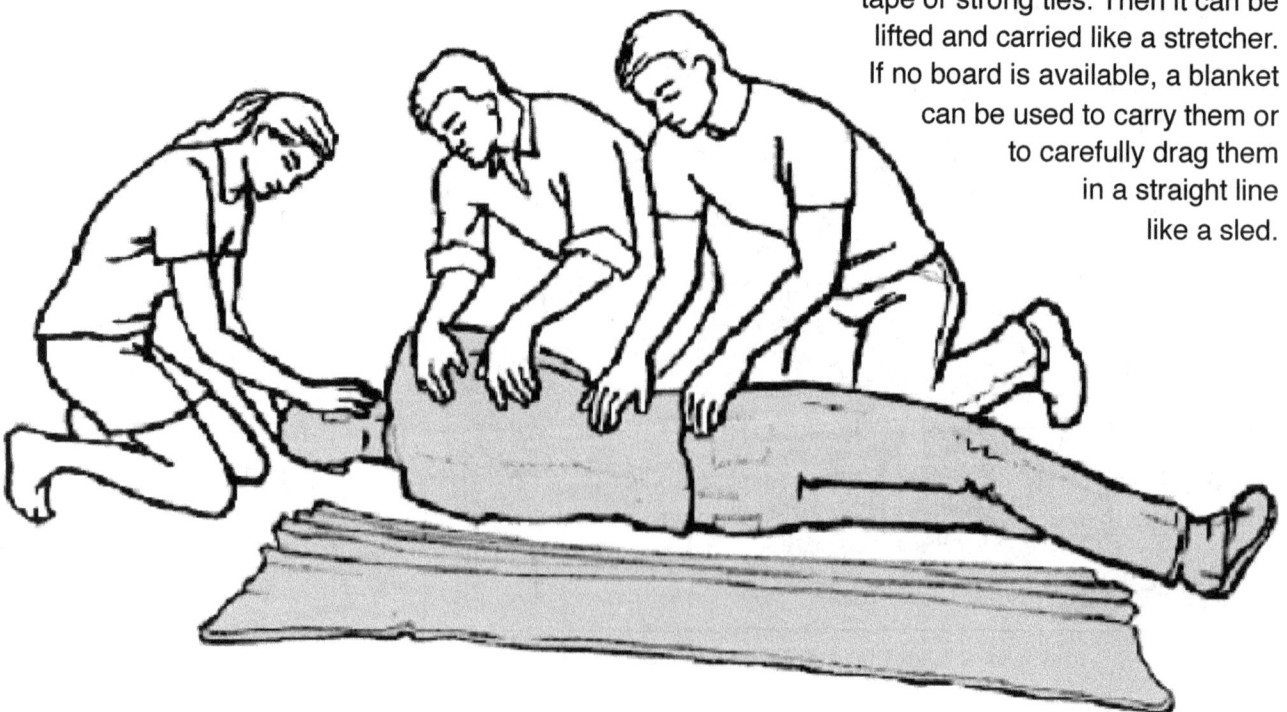

Moving the injured

DON'T HUMP YOUR BACK
Dangerous to your spine!

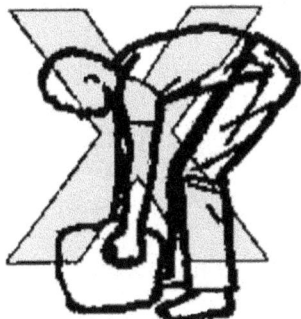

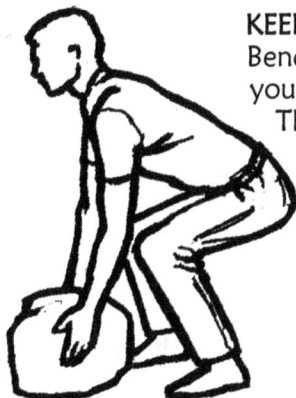

KEEP YOUR BACK STRAIGHT
Bend your knees and lift with your HIP and LEG MUSCLES. These are the largest and strongest muscles of your body.

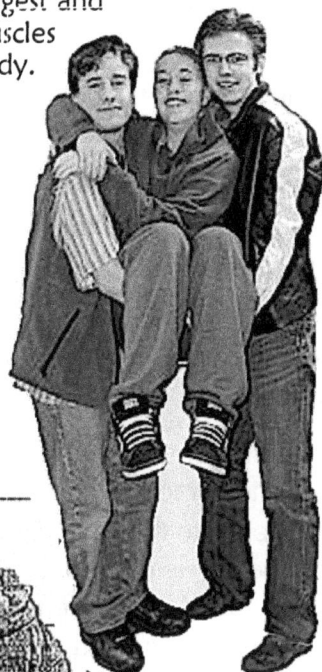

Arm-Seat Carry

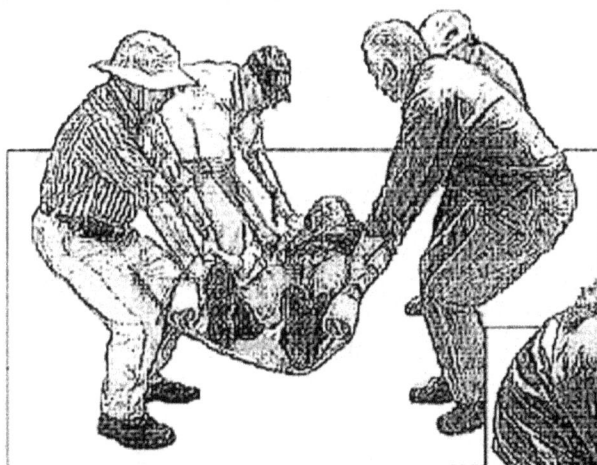

Blanket Lift and Carry

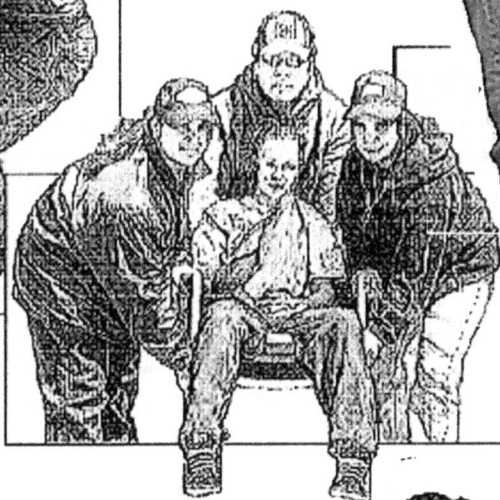

Chair Carry

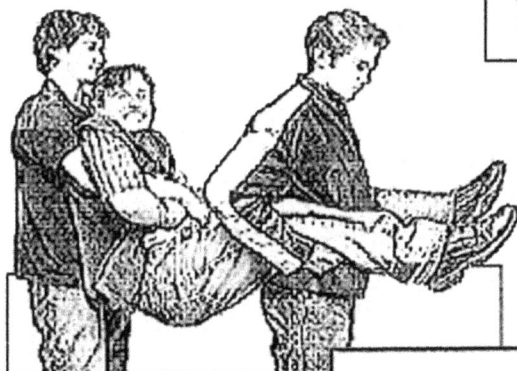

2-Person Carry

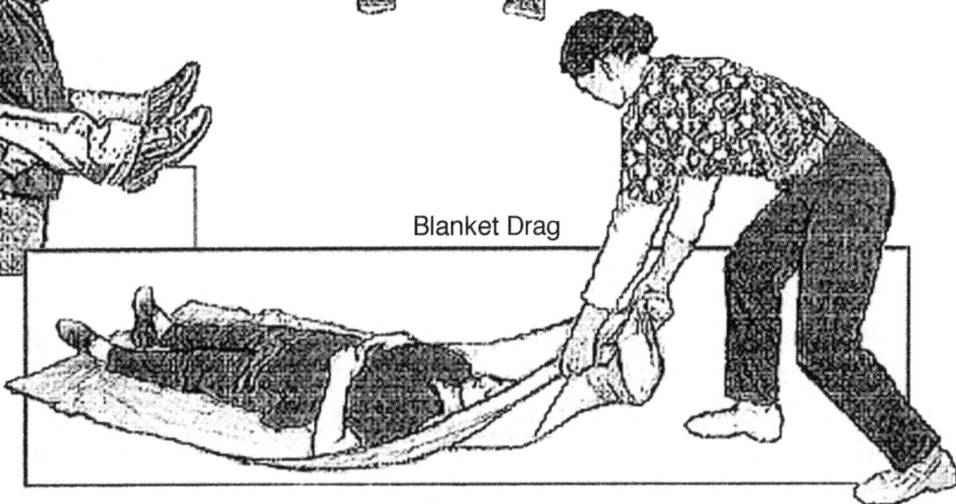

Blanket Drag

QUICK REFERENCE - Treatment Guide

GENERAL

Most closed injuries should be treated with cold packs if possible, on and off 10 to 20 minutes at a time for first 2 days. Cold packs and elevation help to decrease bleeding, swelling, and pain.

OPEN INJURIES, CUTS, ABRASIONS (p.20-21)

Control bleeding, then wash, dry, and bandage the wound. If a splint or sling is also needed, write on the outside of it "open wound." If possible wear rubber or vinyl gloves to protect yourself from blood or body fluids.

BRUISES (p.20)

Cold packs help decrease swelling and pain. NOTE: If bruising is found on the abdomen, chest, or neck, suspect deeper injury and treat preventively for shock. (p.18)

CRUSH INJURY (p.24-25)

Keep the person quiet not active. If the crush injury is to a limb, elevate it and apply cold packs if possible. If any injury to the chest, abdomen, or large areas of limbs, also treat for shock. (p.18)

POSSIBLE SHOCK (p.18)

Have the person lie down. Elevate the legs to higher than their heart level. If there is a head injury, elevate the head also. Conserve normal body heat, including the head. Protect the airway. If the person is nauseous, semi- or completely unconscious, turn them on their side to to keep the airway open, not blocked by the tongue, and to prevent choking or aspirating fluids into the lungs. Do not give them food, fluids or anything by mouth. Send for medical help. (p.14)

FRACTURES AND SPRAINS (p.22)

Stabilize the injured area with splints or wraps to prevent movement and decrease pain. Use soft materials next to the skin, and stiff materials for splints or support. (p.26-27) For arm, shoulder or collarbone use a sling and swath. For leg or hip, support with board splints. If none are available, place padding between the legs and secure both legs to each other for support. The unhurt leg acts as a brace for the injured one.

HEAD, NECK, AND BACK (p. 28)

Do not move the injured person unless there is immediate danger such as fire or other hazard. Be careful not to twist or bend the neck or back. After stabilizing the neck, get enough help, (at least three people) and LOG-ROLL the injured person onto a stretcher (a door, shutter, ironing board) before moving them. Stabilize the neck and back in a straight line, prop with rolled towels, and secure the entire person onto the board with tape or straps to be sure they don't fall off when the board is lifted and carried.

BURNS (p. 23)

Stop the burning process by cooling the burn area with clean water or wet cloths for 10 to 15 minutes. After cooling, remove the wet cloths and cover the burns loosely with clean dry bandages. If there are blisters, DON'T break them. DO NOT apply oils or ointments.

Electrical Burns: DO NOT TOUCH the person until you're absolutely sure the electric source has been TURNED OFF AND REMOVED from them. Check for breathing.

The Days That Follow

The injured have now been identified and treated in your Medical Area and some of the "walking wounded" (people with minor injuries or none) are attending them. Now you should sit down with your group and make some plans for water, shelter, food, and sanitation. (p.40-41)

Clean drinking water is the most essential necessity for sustaining life. Shelter from heat and cold is next in importance. Food is third. It is possible to live without food for several weeks, but human beings can only survive for a few days without water. Shelter helps prevent medical complications from environmental exposure, such as heat stroke, heat exhaustion, or hypothermia (serious loss of core body warmth). (p.34-35)

Things to do in the days that follow

Set up shelters outside if houses are unsafe. Make a shared cooking area out in the open in a fire-safe area. Arrange for some method of hand-washing before handling food.

NEVER use charcoal or camp stoves inside a house or tent or any enclosed space. There is the double danger of carbon monoxide poisoning as well as fire.

Set up a "M.A.S.H." type Medical Aid Area and move the inured there together to make it easier to take care of them. Arrange for sanitation and infection control. Set up a toilet area separated from the living areas. Dispose of wastes properly and carefully to avoid disease.

Re-check, clean, and re-bandage wounds each day, or teach helpers or the injured persons how to do it for themselves. Re-check circulation in all limbs that you have bandaged or splinted. Check & adjust splint ties and bandages as needed. Set up a Morgue area if needed, and notify Police or City authorities if there are any deceased at your location. (p.33).

Things to do NOW - Before the emergency comes

Organize your household or workplace resources. Store water (two gallons of water per day per person, for 3 days or more) and food. Have a sleeping bag for each person. Make up a First Aid Kit and keep it in your car, your home, your office, where it is easily available at all times.

Meet with your neighbors or coworkers. Organize a neighborhood, school, or workplace Rescue Team. Take some Disaster Preparedness classes together from your city or county Fire or Police Dept. Most are free. A group can work together in gathering the essential equipment and medical supplies for first aid kits. Buying in bulk is much less expensive.

Gather information from your city or county Offices of Emergency Services, Fire Departments, and public libraries. Customize your planning to fit your specific needs and situation.

You cannot predict every possibility, but being basically prepared will make a positive difference when an emergency comes. In the meantime, having this knowledge and preparation gives you a degree of confidence and peace of mind.

Infection Control and Sanitation

A soon as practical after the event, fill some containers with tap water. It's likely that a major quake or explosion will rupture water mains and pipes, and the water supply may become contaminated and unsafe. The water in your water heater is safe to drink, but turn off the inlet pipe so no new (contaminated) water will enter. Water in your toilet tank (not toilet bowl) can be used for pets.

Use your cleanest (or bottled) water for drinking and wound cleaning. If you have clean but somewhat less-certain water, it can be disinfected with chlorine bleach. Use about ONE HALF-TEASPOON PER GALLON of water or about 4 DROPS PER QUART. This can be used for hand washing in a bucket set aside for this purpose. Don't use standing water or runoff water, because of the high risk of contamination.

Hands can carry bacteria that spread infection and disease. Wash your hands before and after each injured person you treat, before handling food, and after using the latrine or toilet.

Avoid direct handling of blood or other body fluids and secretions. Wear gloves if possible to protect yourself from blood-borne infectious diseases such as hepatitis, staph, strep, HIV, and others. Unbroken skin is a fairly good barrier, but rubber or vinyl gloves are better.

You should have gloves in your First Aid kit (p.36) but if you have none, you could use plastic bags like mittens for some protection. If nothing else, even non-porous paper or tinfoil may give some protection. Disposable rubber or vinyl gloves can be bought in drugstores, hardware stores, and grocery stores. Or heavier household rubber gloves can be worn and washed off with soap and water before and after treating each injured person.

Basic Sanitation

Normal sanitation services may be damaged or shut down. Improper disposal of human waste and fluids can create serious health problems and spread disease. Set up a toilet area that is away from your living area and Medical Aid area. It should be either LEVEL with these areas or DOWNHILL from them– Not uphill from you – because rain or underground seepage will carry waste products down into your living area.

One method to handle the problem of human waste is to make a LATRINE. Dig a trench that's at least 2 feet long, 6 inches wide, and at least 2 feet deep - deeper if possible. After each use of the latrine, take a small scoop of dry powdered household bleach or powdered agricultural lime (available in garden supply and hardware stores) and sprinkle it directly over the waste. Then sprinkle a scoop of dirt on top. Lime is caustic (can cause chemical burns). Avoid getting it on your hands or clothing. When done, wash your hands.

Infection Control and Sanitation

Or you can make a good temporary TOILET from a sturdy small trash can with a tight fitting lid. Line the container with two heavy-duty plastic bags, one inside the other. Then place a layer of absorbent material such as shredded newspaper or kitty-litter into the inside bag. After using the toilet, sprinkle dry powdered bleach or lime onto the waste. Use minimal toilet paper and put it into the bag also. Replace the cover carefully so that nothing leaks or spills.

When the container is two-thirds full, twist and tie the inner bag, then twist and tie the outer bag too. Then remove this from the container and bury it in a latrine that is away from, downwind, and level or downhill from your living and medical care areas.

Morgue

Unfortunately but realistically, some lives may be lost due to circumstances beyond your control. If you have any deceased at your location, report this to your communications point (nearest Fire Station) as early as possible. They may be able to arrange for the proper removal of the deceased. If not, they can give you instructions for what to do.

Generally it is appropriate to cover the deceased respectfully and leave them where they were found if you know that authorities are coming soon. Your first concern at this time is for the living, and what you can do to help them.

However if no help will be available for a period of hours or days, the deceased should be moved to a morgue area that is some distance from your living area and medical area. Plan the placement of the morgue area carefully, taking into consideration elements such as wind, weather, and privacy. An appropriate location would be a place that is as cool and dry as possible, downwind, level or downhill from your living area, and accessible to Emergency vehicles.

EXPOSURE: The Environmental

After an earthquake, explosion, or fire, many buildings may be unsafe. You may have to live, work, and sleep outdoors, at risk for environmental dangers such as Exposure to heat and cold. The risk of HEAT EXHAUSTION or HEAT STROKE is increased by strenuous work, hot weather, or humidity.

The injured are at greater risk for HYPOTHERMIA (dangerous LOSS of body heat) especially if they must sit or lie on the ground. The best plan will be to avoid the complications of both heat and cold exposure by taking preventive measures.

PREVENT Heat Exhaustion and Heat Stroke

- DRINK WATER about every 15 to 20 minutes before, during, and after physical activity. Avoid dehydration by replacing fluids often. Don't wait until you are thirsty.

- WEAR A HAT. Cover the back of your neck and shoulders. Avoid sunburn. Wear loose-fitting, light-colored clothes. Rest in the shade when you get tired or become overheated.

- RECOGNIZE SYMPTOMS of heat illness and take action promptly.

Heat Exhaustion looks like this:

- Skin is sweaty, may be pale, cool, and clammy.
- Weakness and fatigue, muscle cramping.
- Pulse rapid and "bounding" at first, then becoming weaker or thready.
- Headache, often with nausea.
- Dizziness, impaired judgment.
- May or MAY NOT feel thirsty.

What To Do

1. Move the person to shade or a cool place.
2. Check breathing, circulation, & mental status.
3. Remove clothes and sponge body with cool (not cold) water.
4. If fully conscious, give cool water to sip.

5. DO NOT GIVE SALT! Sports drink DILUTED 50-50 with water okay.
6. DO NOT give full-strength sports drinks, fruit juices or cola/soft drinks! These delay absorption of water into the bloodstream.

Heat Exhaustion may progress to Heat Stroke:

- Skin appears red, feels either hot and dry, or hot and damp. In late stages, sweating may stop.
- Mental status is altered. May be confused, or irrational, or groggy, or may become unconscious.
- Heat Stroke may be accompanied by seizures. Severe Heat Stroke can cause death.

What To Do - GET MEDICAL HELP

1. Move the person to shade or a cool place.
2. Remove clothes and sponge their body with cool water and fan continuously.
3. Apply ice packs to head and neck, armpits, and groin (pulse points).

4. Stop aggressive cooling when oral temperature drops below 102 degrees.
5. If fully conscious and not vomiting, give sips of cold water. DO NOT give fruit juice, colas or sports drinks. DO NOT GIVE SALT!

Hazards of Heat and Cold

HYPOTHERMIA is the dangerous loss of adequate body-core heat. It can occur even without very cold weather. Being outdoors for long periods of time, wearing wet clothing, sitting or sleeping on the ground – all can cause rapid loss of essential body heat. Infants and children, the elderly, and the ill or injured are at greatest risk. Severe hypothermia can cause death.

PREVENT Hypothermia

- PROTECT THE INJURED from direct contact with the ground. Place plastic sheeting, then a layer of cardboard, crumpled newspapers, or leaves, then blankets or sleeping bags.

- DRESS IN LAYERS. Add on or take off as weather conditions change.

- STAY DRY. If the inside layer of clothing gets wet with sweat, replace it with dry.

- WRAP UP to minimize body heat loss. Have a lightweight water repellent jacket, hat and gloves. Army surplus wool hats and gloves are excellent. (Wool and silk will still keep you warm even when wet.) Cover your head and also the heads of the injured.

- WEAR HARD-SOLED SHOES OR BOOTS to protect your feet from broken glass, metal, etc, with wool socks if possible to help maintain your body heat.

Early Hypothermia looks like this:

Shivering, slow or slurred speech. Altered mental states such as sleepy, poor judgement, confused, silly or inappropriate emotions. May have stumbling or unsteady walk.

What to do

1. Remove wet clothing and place the person in a dry warm sleeping bag, well insulated from the ground, and in a wind-proof shelter if possible.

2. If conscious, give sips of warm fluids. DO NOT give alcohol, coffee, tea or cola.

3. Handle gently. Do not rub or massage.

SEVERE Hypothermia looks like this:

Cold to the touch, shivering stops, skin looks waxy or blue, mental status is altered, confused, unresponsive or unconscious. Pulse and breathing are slow and faint, hard to detect.

What to do - GET MEDICAL HELP

1. Check breathing, circulation, and mental status. Use the NECK ARTERY to check for pulse, and take more time, because the pulse is likely to be very slow and faint.

2. Handle them very gently. Carefully avoid bumping while moving them to a warm sheltered area.

3. Warm the person gradually. Remove their clothes and place them in a warmed sleeping bag, or get into the sleeping bag with them and warm them with your body heat.

4. Do not use high heat devices such as electric blankets. But you can heat some dry towels and place them at the head, neck, armpits, and groin pulse points.

5. DO NOT attempt to give anything by mouth unless the person is fully conscious and able to sit up and swallow without choking. DO NOT give alcohol, coffee, tea, or cola.

First Aid Kits & Supplies

"Store-bought" First Aid kits are not likely to have what you need for a major emergency because they are intended for minor or temporary situations. We examined dozens of expensive commercial First Aid kits, advertised on the internet as being "for disaster." We found that NONE of them would be adequate, consisting of mostly small-sized materials, too few of them, and things like band-aids, aspirin, and candy bars. Advertising and fancy packaging are common. They are not illegal, but they can be very misleading. It's better (and cheaper) to build your own first aid kit if possible.

Get a sturdy nylon or canvas bag that's big enough, water-resistant, and has lots of easy-to-reach pockets. A bright color is good. (Or you can "roll-your-own" using the diagram on p.38-39.) Then stock it with the supplies and materials you actually need.

Your First Aid Kit for Earthquake and Disaster must be more than the ordinary kit. It should have bigger-sized materials and more of them. Your kit should be compact, well stocked, kept up to date, and easy to reach quickly, in your home, workplace, or car. Here's a list of basic essentials. Use it to get started, then add your specific personal or group needs to the list.

Suggested Supplies for your Disaster First Aid Kit

- This Disaster First Aid Handbook
- Tags & marking pens for Rapid Triage
- Latex or vinyl gloves, 20 to 50 pairs
- Cloth adhesive tapes 1" and 2" wide (3 each)
- Plastic adhesive tapes 1" and 2" wide (3 each)
- Large sterile gauze dressings 6" x10" (10 or 12)
- Extra-Large band-aids 2"x 4" or larger
- Box of sanitary napkins (these make good absorbent dressings or pressure dressings)
- 2 Large packs (of 100) non-sterile 4"x4"gauze (good for controlling bleeding & misc.)
- Rolled bandages (Kling or Kerlix, or make your own from strips of washed old sheets p.37)
- Triangle "cravat" slings (or make your own)
- Tongue depressors and cotton swabs
- Lots of extra-large safety pins
- Liquid disinfectant Green Soap or Betadine scrub
- 2% Hydrogen Peroxide (to be diluted with water)
- Antibiotic ointment (Polysporin, Bacitracin, etc.)
- Sterile saline (for wound cleaning/ eye flushing)

- Large waterproof Magic Markers
- First Report and Second Report forms
- Clipboard tablet and pens
- Plastic baggies and heavy garbage bags
- Plastic sheeting ground cover 12x25 ft.roll
- Mylar "space blankets" (6 or more)
- clothesline-type rope or sash-cord
- "Duck" Tape (good for everything)
- Blunt-ended "EMT" scissors (2 or 3 pairs)
- Kitchen rubber gloves for general mess
- Pocket knife or folding lock-blade knife
- Clean plastic squirt bottle or spray bottle for cleaning wounds with a spray of water.
- Keep 2 weeks supply of any prescription medications you or family usually take (changed monthly to keep them fresh)
- Tylenol or aspirin for FEVER (Remember that aspirin can increase bleeding)
- Anti-Diarrhea medicine (if possible seek medical advice before using medications)

Then add whatever else you think you'll need for yourself, your family, your workplace.

First Aid Kits & Supplies

We encourage "outside the box" resourcefulness and practical creative thinking. Learn to use whatever you have, and you will always find what you need, no matter where you are. Prepare some homemade supplies in advance. Rolls of bandages can be made from strips of old sheets. These are going to be the outer wrapping that doesn't touch the wound, so they don't have to be sterilized. Just wash the material in hot water with a good dose of chlorine bleach (an effective disinfectant). After drying, tear into strips for splint ties and bandages, and cut some triangles of material for arm slings. Pillow cases also make great slings. Copy the Triage Tag onto heavy card-stock, then cut apart, hole-punch, and add a string or large safety pin to each and put them into your first aid kit.

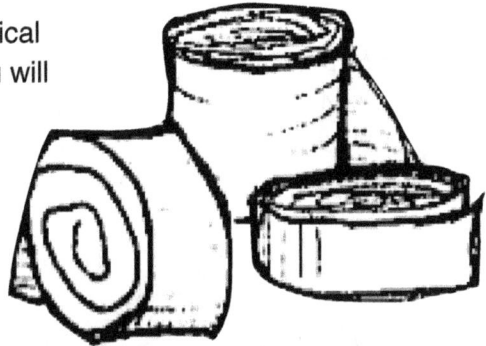

Have Fun Making Your Own First Aid Supplies

Why not have a potluck, or a neighborhood meeting and enjoy some socializing? While everybody tears the sheet material into strips of different widths, (kids enjoy this) then roll them into different sized rolls. Store them in ziplock baggies for individuals, families, or your neighborhood group's Disaster Preparedness Team first aid kit. They make excellent splint ties, bandage wrapping, and are handy for all sorts of things from controlling bleeding to repairing tents. Getting to know your neighbors a little better is practical as well as social. When any serious emergency happens, you will need them, and they will need you.

THE CLASSIC TRIANGLE SLING

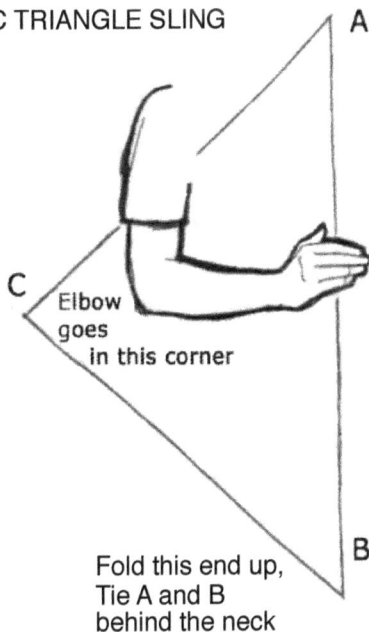

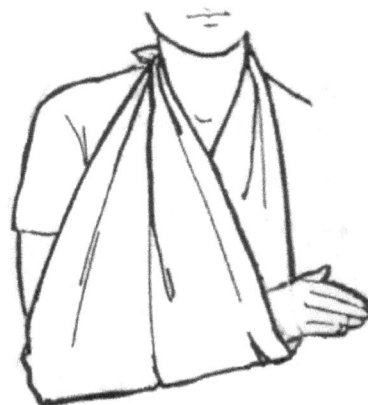

A

C

Elbow
goes
in this corner

B

Fold this end up,
Tie A and B
behind the neck

You can make this sling out of almost anything, old sheets cut into triangles, or a scarf folded in half becomes a triangle. More ideas and innovations are on page 27, pillowcase sling and T-shirt sling & swath.

Roll-Your-Own

The finished bag should be about 2 ft. x 4 ft. or 3 ft. x 5 ft. Fabric for the outside should be heavy-gauge water-resistant back-pack material with straps made of nylon webbing. The inside pockets can be clear vinyl or mesh see-through material. Add elastic bands for bigger items. Sew with nylon thread, or waxed thread if you can get it. This is not a precise pattern, but a rough diagram to get you started. You're welcome to adapt it and develop your own best design.

HERE'S WHAT IT LOOKS LIKE WHEN IT'S DONE

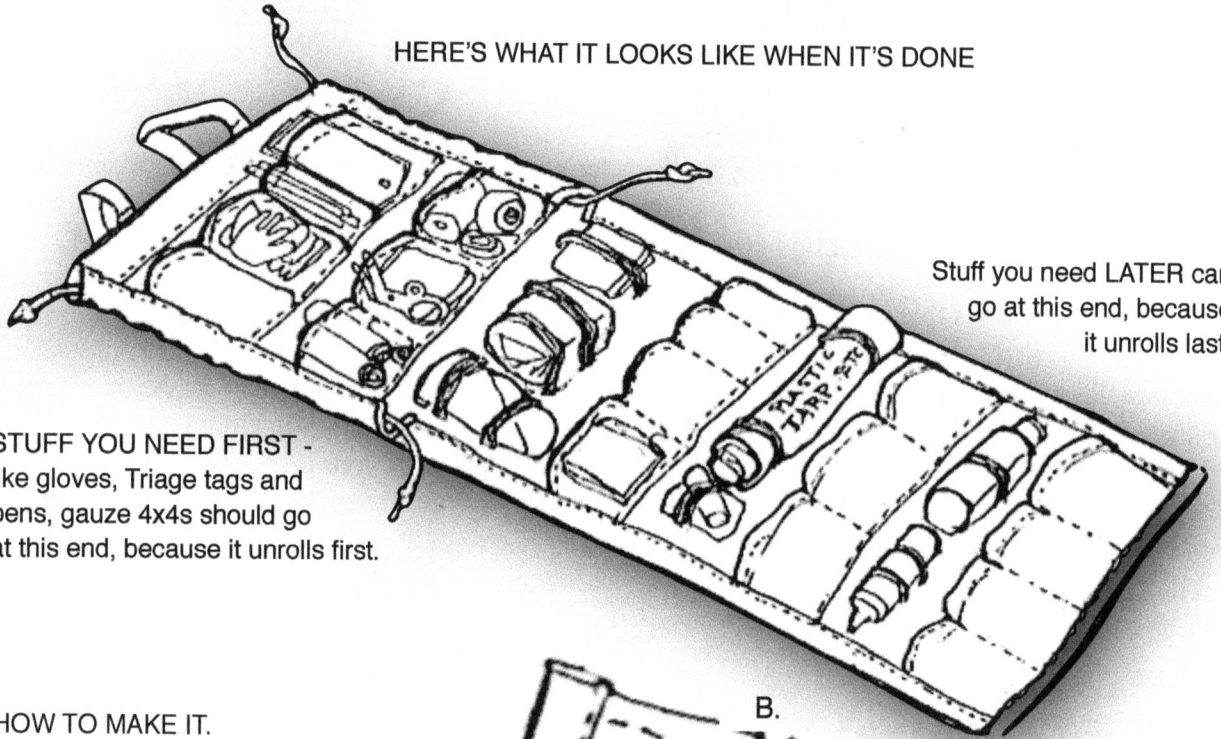

Stuff you need LATER can go at this end, because it unrolls last.

STUFF YOU NEED FIRST - like gloves, Triage tags and pens, gauze 4x4s should go at this end, because it unrolls first.

HOW TO MAKE IT.

1. Turn down about 2 or 3 inches at the top edge (marked A) and stitch. Your carrying strap will go here later.

2. Make a notch about 18 to 24 inches below the top edge on each side (B) for the drawstring to exit. Sew a border of extra material around the notch to strengthen it. It will look like this.

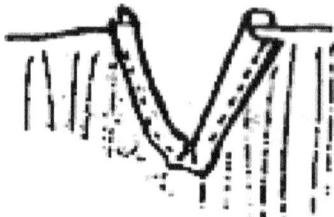

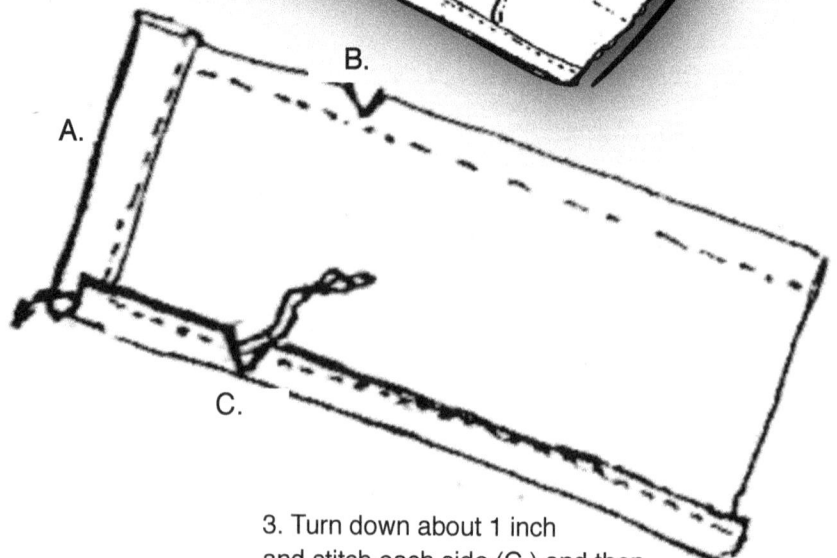

A.

B.

C.

3. Turn down about 1 inch and stitch each side (C.) and then Run the drawstring cord through the upper section. Now it looks like this.

First Aid Kit-Bag

This type of First Aid kit has several advantages. You can drag it behind you like a sled if you have to go some distances between the injured people you're helping, or in your set-up Medical Area you can use the straps at the top to hang the open bag on a tree or tent in your Medical Area, so your first aid supplies are all visible and easy to reach.

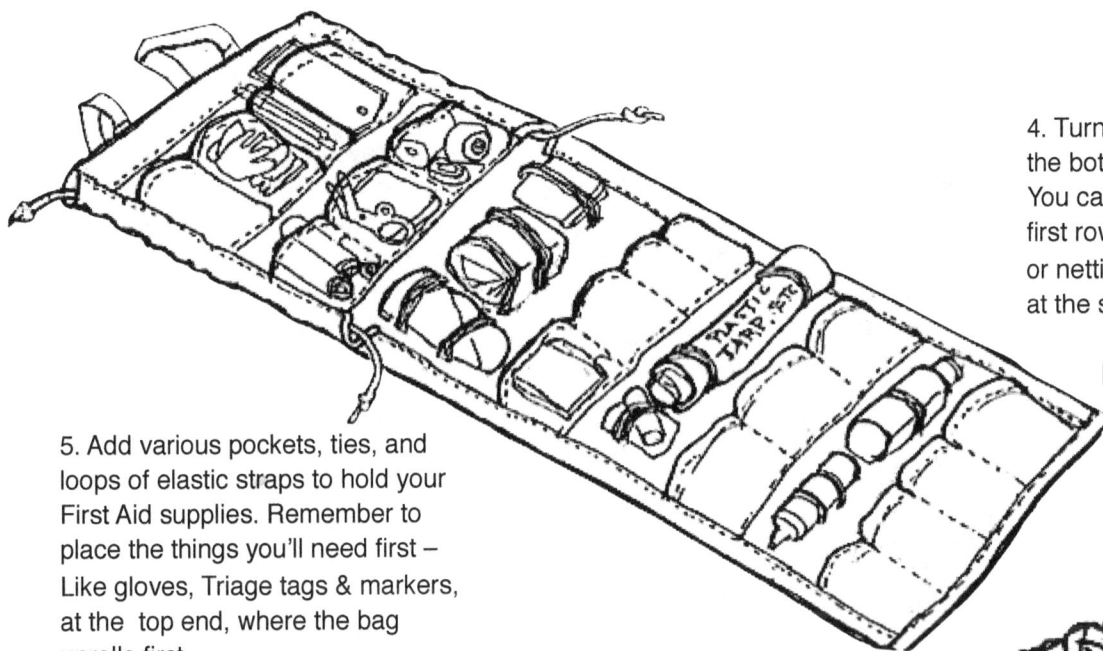

4. Turn up and stitch the bottom edge (D.) You can include the first row of your plastic or netting pockets at the same time.

D.

5. Add various pockets, ties, and loops of elastic straps to hold your First Aid supplies. Remember to place the things you'll need first – Like gloves, Triage tags & markers, at the top end, where the bag unrolls first.

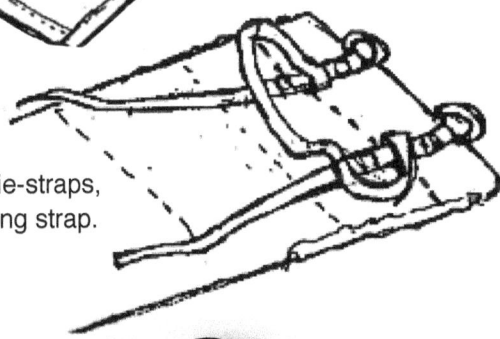

6. Add the roll-up tie-straps, tie-rings and carrying strap.

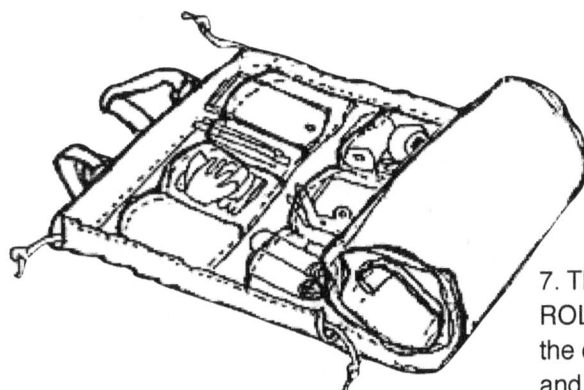

7. Then Fill it up, ROLL it up, tie the drawstrings and GO.

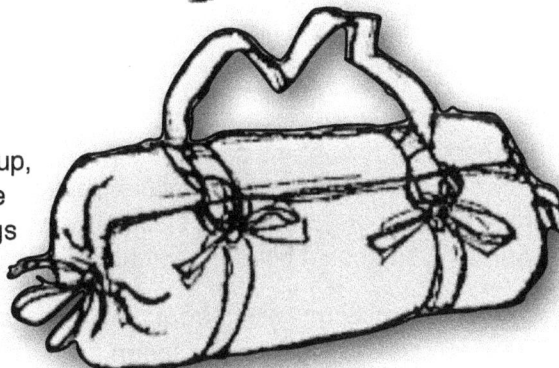

After the Disaster, Surviving

AFTER EARTHQUAKES, hurricanes, tsunamis, floods, volcanoes, mud slides and other disasters, the people who survived the original events find themselves faced with another disaster, a kind of "urban wilderness" even in in cities, without clean water, groceries, electricity, sanitation, and in many cases without shelter from sun and rain, heat and cold. Here are some ideas to help you survive the problems that come after the disaster.

In the days that followed the Katrina hurricane, the damage was not over. People were tossed out into the floodplain unprepared. Many died in the floods, but even more shocking was the fact that about three hundred people died from dehydration and related problems because they did not have clean water. And yet there was plenty of water in every home before the storm hit, and 4 full days of warning that the storm was coming. They could have prepared by drawing up drinking water into bottles, buckets, and other containers. But they didn't. In every disaster, many people die innocently and needlessly because they don't know what to do, or because they expect outside help to come quickly and save everyone. Tragically, we now know that very often this is impossible. The sheer numbers and logistics (such as roads blocked, bridges down, 911 emergency Medical services overwhelmed) usually make it impossible to do enough, fast enough, to save everybody.

Even though many people may be lost no matter what, hundreds will also die who didn't have to. They could have been saved, or saved themselves, if only they had known what to do. At Disaster First Aid we believe that whatever can be done, should be done, to prevent loss of life or limbs whenever possible. So we have researched and found some simple actions anyone can do for themselves and others to cope with medical emergencies and post-disaster problems and dangers. Here are some of those things. These ideas are by no means complete, but they are the barest essentials of easily do-able actions that all of us need to know in order to survive not only the disaster but also the difficulties and dangers of the days that will follow.

1. Water is the most important physical necessity to sustain life. The human body is made up of about 80% water, and every single cell of the body must have enough of it at all times. Through natural functions like sweating, breathing, and passing off the body's waste products, some water is being lost all the time. It must be constantly replaced, usually by drinking water. Things like fruit juice, cola, and sport drinks don't do the same job that water does, and because they contain sugar and salt, they actually increase thirst, delay absorption, and worsen heat-related illnesses like heat exhaustion and heat stroke. When body fluid levels get too low (dehydration) a series of events are set in motion, interfering with the blood's essential needs, nutrients, and electrolytes. This causes rising body temperatures, weakness and dizziness, hyperthermia (heat illness) and may set off some heart dysrhythmias. Water is life-giving.

It must be CLEAN. Unclean water carries bacteria that cause diarrhea and vomiting which worsen dehydration, and over time can result in severe weakness and even death. Instead: Put up and store clean water in sturdy plastic (not glass) containers in your home, car, or workplace. Use 2 drops of chlorine bleach per gallon to disinfect tap water for storage. Later, if you have to use other water you're not sure of, you should boil it first before drinking it or using it on an open wound.

2. Shelter. Protecting yourself from cold, heat, and wetness helps prevent many problems from post-disaster conditions, such as hypothermia (loss of essential body-core heat) and hyperthermia (heat exhaustion and heat stroke). After an earthquake, choose a shelter location in an open area away from tall buildings with glass windows and away from any structure or large tree, or power lines that may fall onto you. When you look for a location, remember to look up. Consider a parking lot. An open park with cooking grills and only small trees might be ideal. NEVER light any fire, grill, or heater, INSIDE a closed space, tent, or shelter! There is the double danger of fire and carbon monoxide poisoning. Tents are great if you have one, but you can also make a simple shelter out of a tarp, blanket, or plastic garden sheeting thrown over low shrubs or bushes, then crawl in underneath. Living plants have heat of their own, which helps you stay warm. You can buy "tube tents" for yourself and your family members (a heavyweight plastic tube about 6 feet long, wide enough for one person and sleeping bag. Most camping and surplus stores have them. Or make a "clothesline tent" by tying a rope between two objects (ie. the "clothesline") and then throwing a tarp, a mylar "space blanket" or some heavy plastic sheeting over it and staking the corners to the ground. (Like you did in the back yard when you were 10 years old.) An excellent source of ideas for more emergency shelters can be found in the Boy Scout Handbook, available in bookstores and at your local public library.

3. Personal protection. In COLD or cool weather keep warm and dry. Wear layers, cover your head, hands, and feet. Wool is best because it still keeps you warm even if wet. If you don't have gloves, put socks on your hands. Wear a hat, a paper bag, or thick plastic granny-scarf. (Never put thin cling-able plastic on children! It is a suffocation hazard). To sleep when blankets are scarce, try "dog-piling," an effective way to share warmth Invented by our caveman ancestors. Insulate yourself from the ground. Place plastic sheeting, then a mat of leaves, newspapers, or branches under your sleeping bag.

RAIN: If you don't have a raincoat but you do have heavy plastic garden sheeting (a roll should be kept with your First Aid kit) just cut a piece about 8 to 10 feet long (or twice the height from your neck to your knees) and about 6 feet wide (or twice the length from your neck to your hand). Then cut a hole right in the middle and stick your head through. Instant Parka!

HEAT. Work in the coolest time of the morning and evening and rest in the hottest part of the day. Use light colors for your clothes and tents if possible because they reflect light and don't absorb much heat. In cold weather, just the opposite, dark-colors will gather some heat to last after sunset.

4. Food. This is the least important thing in the first few days. Though you will be hungry, a normally healthy person can survive for up to 3 weeks without food and still fully recover, but remember you can only go about 2 days without water. When you put aside your emergency drinking water, also put aside some canned or packaged foods that can be eaten without cooking. Canned beans,vegetables, meats and fish are good, powdered milk is a good source of protein. Also mylar-wrapped nutrition bars like granola bars and "Cliff" bars. Read the labels. Make sure you're not just getting candy or cookies with an athletic-sounding name. Date everything with a magic-marker and replace your stashed food with new, every few months.

5. Keep well, keep safe. It's extremely important to get enough rest and sleep, even in a disaster, to keep your strength going. Drink water frequently and eat at natural times if possible. You may be tempted to just keep working, but if you do, you will soon burn out. Fatigue increases your risk of accidents and injury. Work with a group, and tag-team frequent time-outs for everyone to get rest and water. Watch for signs of fatigue, heat exhaustion, or hypothermia in each other. Keeping yourself as well and as safe as you can is a serious responsibility. You can't help anyone else if you get injured, or weakened by dehydration. Always put your own safety FIRST. That's how you will be most able to help others.

Reprinted by permission from Life Lines article "Surviving the Urban Wilderness, www.DisasterFirstAid.com

Epilogue

There are major earthquake faults all across the U.S. and throughout the world. Essentially, wherever there is a mountain range or a valley, there is an old fault line, as well as unmarked ones on land and offshore beneath the oceans. The fact of the matter is, the earth itself is alive, and will move at times. The National Geological Survey states that there is a 70% probability of a massive earthquake in California that could occur at any time. And of course, terrorism and mass-casualty violence is also happening worldwide. An unexpected major emergency is a real possibility, right now, and even right where you are.

In a major disaster there may be hundreds or even thousands of people injured. There simply will not be enough medical help and rescue for everyone at once. After the Loma Prieta earthqake of 1989, most U.S. state and federal disaster response agencies formally warned that in any mass-casualty emergency, the great majority of us must expect to be "on our own" for at least 24 hours to 3 days or longer until more help can be brought from other areas.

Yet we may need to take action immediately in order to save ourselves and others in those critical first minutes, hours, and days when the most lives are either saved or lost, including the many that could have been saved with simple measures, if done soon after the injury, before they worsen over the time of waiting for help. In the first hours and days, we may have to rely on our own good common sense and our own two hands.

A Study by the American College of Trauma Surgeons researched three types of trauma deaths:

Type 1 –Death in minutes from overwhelming damage to body and vital organs. (cannot be saved)

Type 2 –Death within several hours from severe bleeding or shock. (might have been saved if...)

Type 3 –Death in days or weeks from infection, organ failure, shock.(might have been saved if...)

This study estimated that of those who had a chance to survive (Type 2 and Type 3) but died, as many as 40% of these could have been saved by simple First Aid measures, IF they had been received EARLY, or within the "Golden Hour" after the injury occurred.

Time Is Life

Now You Have the Basic Tools. In this book you have learned the essential information and skills needed to be able to prevent the preventable deaths, and to care for and prevent worsening of injuries while waiting for medical help. You have a foundation of knowledge of What To Do, When, and How. You know how to think "outside the box" and to improvise actions and materials.

Knowledge is powerful., and ltimately what's in your mind will be more important than what's in your First Aid Kit. What's in your mind is always with you, anywhere and any time, even in unexpected situations. Though you may not be experienced at the task at hand, having this essential knowledge enables you to make sound decisions and take appropriate actions,

In a Medical Crisis, Time is often the deciding factor between life or death. A significant number of lives can be "saved" just by preventing the injury from worsening, or sometimes just by helping someone to maintain hope and the will to live. You could make the critical difference.

REFERENCES and INFORMATION SOURCES

Alameda County California Emergency Medical Services
Policy and Procedures Manual:
Policy #8070 Medical Management of Multi-Casualty Incidents
Policy #8073 S.T.A.R.T. Triage
Policy #8210 Trauma Patient Evaluation

Multi-Casualty Incident Scene Management Plan
Alameda County Fire Chiefs' Association EMS Section

Basic Trauma Life Support, 2nd Edition
John Emory Campbell, MD

Alabama Chapter American College of Emergency Physicians
ISBN: 0-89303-088-0

Emergency Care and Transportation of the Sick and Injured
6th Edition, Instructor Edition

American Academy of Orthopedic Surgeons
ISBN: 0-7637-076-1

More than 25 years of first-hand experience
as a Fire Department First-Responder and
hospital E.R. Emergency Medical Caregiver

There's More You Can Do:

Teach Disaster First Aid where you live

For your neighborhood or your employee safety program at work. The DFA course only takes one day, and these common-sense techniques can be taught by nonprofessionals and learned and practiced by anyone from age 14 to seniors. You don't need to be a professional teacher. Citizen disaster team leaders can teach it in their own neighborhoods, and Employers can teach it in the workplace as part of their Disaster Preparedness and Homeland Security programs.

EMTs, paramedics, firefighters, and nurses, but also coaches, camp counselors, Eagle Scouts, scoutmasters, den-mothers, and others can teach DFA for their community, and the course can also be taught as a small business. FAQs and information for instructors are available at our website: www.disasterfirstaid.com, or email: support@disasterfirstaid.com

Ask for DFA to be taught at your school

Will your children be taken care of, if an earthquake or another disaster happens while they are at school? In large emergencies, standard first aid will be inadequate. Schools are teaching this Disaster First aid to their faculty and administrators, and many of them are teaching their high schools and middle school students as well. DFA is a condensed course of life-saving information and skills that anyone can learn in one day, yet it has more of what you actually need for disaster than Standard or Advanced first aid courses that take weeks or months.

Request DFA from your city or County Disaster Preparedness Program

This course is often used by C.E.R.T. Programs, because it has been designed to interface with Fire and Police Department public education programs, and DFA is based on the same standard practices and protocols used by these public safety agencies for multi-casual emergencies, scaled down and adapted to the citizens level of ability and resources.

The Instructor Kit / Teaching Manual and Materials includes: Instructor Guide / Manual, DFA handbook, Teaching Outline, copymaster forms for class administration (liability releases, student handouts, worksheets) Instructor Task checklist and supplies & equipment checklist, ISBN #0-9714359-8-7 The Instructor package also includes the PowerPoint Teaching Presentation of 80 detailed color slides for PC and Mac, ISBN 978-0-9714359-9-5 The Instructor package is available ONLY through the website. Contact: Support@disasterfirstaid.com

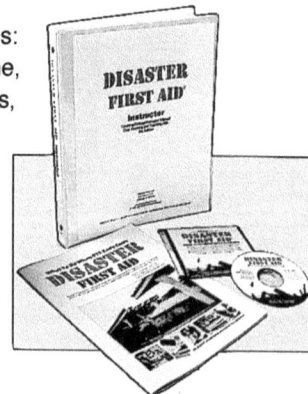

Please Support your local bookstore. Disaster First Aid handbooks are available from Barnes and Noble, Amazon, and Ingram, but any brick-and-mortar bookstore can also order it for you. You'll save time and money this way since there's no delivery charge to pay. Help us save Real bookstores and Real books. Thank you!

www.ingramcontent.com/pod-product-compliance
Lightning Source LLC
Chambersburg PA
CBHW080926050426
42334CB00055B/2830